Pulmonary and Respiratory Diseases and Disorders

nova
Medicine & Health
New York

Pulmonary and Respiratory Diseases and Disorders

Understanding and Treating Acute Pulmonary Embolism
James K. Edwards (Editor)
2022. ISBN: 979-8-88697-149-1 (Softcover)
2022. ISBN: 979-8-88697-398-3 (eBook)

Chronic Obstructive Pulmonary Disease: From Diagnosis to Treatment
Jaber S. Alqahtani, PhD (Editor)
2022. ISBN: 979-8-88697-333-4 (Hardcover)
2022. ISBN: 979-8-88697-396-9 (eBook)

Interstitial Lung Disease: From Diagnosis to Treatment
Roberto G. Carbone, MD, FCCP (Editor)
Francesco Puppo, MD (Editor)
Keith Wille, MD, MSPH (Editor)
Pallav Shah, MD (Editor)
2022. ISBN: 978-1-68507-926-0 (Hardcover)
2022. ISBN: 979-8-88697-068-5 (eBook)

A Clinical Manual of Sarcoidosis
Vikas Pathak, MD (Editor)
Shambhu Aryal, MD (Editor)
2022. ISBN: 978-1-68507-681-8 (Hardcover)
2022. ISBN: 978-1-68507-782-2 (eBook)

Pulmonary Vascular Disorders
Francesco Puppo, MD (Editor),
Roberto G. Carbone, MD, FCCP (Editor),
Victor F. Tapson, MD, FCCP, FRCP (Editor)
2021. ISBN: 978-1-53619-458-6 (Hardcover)
2021. ISBN: 978-1-53619-553-8 (eBook)

More information about this series can be found at
https://novapublishers.com/product-category/series/pulmonary-and-respiratory-diseases-and-disorders/

Antonio M. Esquinas
Dimitrios A. Lagonidis
Pedro Silva Santos
and Bushra Mina
Editors

Nasal High Flow and Non-Invasive Ventilatory Support

Essential Methodology for an Escalation Approach in Respiratory Failure

Medicine & Health
New York

DOI: https://doi.org/10.52305/AVRN8916.

NOTICE TO THE READER

Library of Congress Cataloging-in-Publication Data

Names: Esquinas, Antonio M., editor.
Title: Nasal high flow and non-invasive ventilatory support : essential methodology for an escalation approach in respiratory failure / editors, Antonio M. Esquinas, MD, PHD, FCCP, FAARC, Intensive Care Unit Hospital Morales Meseguer, Murcia, Spain; Director, International School of Non-Invasive Ventilation; Director, International Non Invasive Ventilation Expert of College, Dimitrios A. Lagonidis, MD, PHD, FCCP, Pulmonologist-Intensivist, Director of ICU, Critical Care, Pulmonary and Sleep Medicine Services, Giannitsa General Hospital; Giannitsa, Greece, Pedro Silva Santos, MD, Pulmonology Unit, Centro Hospitalar e Universitário de Coimbra, Hospitais da Universidade de Coimbra, Coimbra, Portugal, Bushra Mina, Pulmonary Critical Care Medicine, Northwell/Lenox Hill Hospital, New York, USA.
Description: New York : Nova Science Publishers, [2023] | Series: Pulmonary and respiratory diseases and disorders | Includes bibliographical references and index. |
Identifiers: LCCN 2023021920 (print) | LCCN 2023021921 (ebook) | ISBN 9798886974201 (hardcover) | ISBN 9798886978902 (adobe pdf)
Subjects: LCSH: Respiratory insufficiency--Treatment. | Respiratory therapy--Equipment and supplies. | Respiratory intensive care--Equipment and supplies.
Classification: LCC RC776.R4 N37 2023 (print) | LCC RC776.R4 (ebook) | DDC 616.2--dc23/eng/20230607
LC record available at https://lccn.loc.gov/2023021920 | LC ebook record available at https://lccn.loc.gov/2023021921

Published by Nova Science Publishers, Inc. † New York

To the authors of this book for their efforts and contributions,
and to all our patients who show us the right path.

Contents

Preface

The non-invasive respiratory support is applied by means of three modalities: High-flow nasal cannula, continuous positive airway pressure (CPAP) and non-invasive ventilation (i.e., pressure-support ventilation with PEEP).

Apart from the management of acute hypoxemic respiratory failure in ICU and the Emergency Department, in the last decade we have witnessed the application of these noninvasive methods in other settings, such as during bronchoscopy and exercise, for domiciliary use and as a palliative care in patients with a Do-Not-Intubate order.

This important development of clinical indications entails being able to define an adequate methodology strategy in order to achieve the fundamental goals of alleviating hypoxemia, of decreasing the work of breathing, of relieving from dyspnea and finally of averting intubation.

However, although these objectives are easy to define, the most perfect approach is unknown. Escalation and de-escalation therapy represent a recent concept, where the clinician defines a clinical situation of progression to higher levels of treatment when the criteria for improvement are not met. However, these aspects are not well established in the literature.

This original book provides the first description in the methodology and approaches in various situations of hypoxemic respiratory failure and the current recommendations to organize the management of these patients.

In non-invasive ventilation escalation and de-escalation therapy approaches, we think that the most important thing is not to have an adequate answer, but to formulate an adequate question in your clinical practice.

Antonio M. Esquinas, MD, PhD
Dimitrios A. Lagonidis, MD
Pedro Silva Santos, MD
Bushra Mina, MD

Chapter 1

Options and Methodology

Arzu Topeli*, MD, MSc

Department of Internal Medicine, Division of Intensive Care,
Hacettepe University Faculty of Medicine, Ankara, Turkey

Abstract

Oxygen (O_2) therapy is essential in both critically ill patients and patients with chronic respiratory failure as long-term O_2 therapy (LTOT). The main indication of O_2 therapy is the prevention and treatment of hypoxemia and tissue hypoxia. Monitorization of O_2 saturation measured by a pulse oximeter (SpO_2) is the most widely used method.

O_2 delivery systems are generally classified as low-flow devices providing a variable fraction of inspired O_2 (FiO_2) or high-flow devices providing fixed FiO_2. The choice of the device is determined by several factors including the clinical status of the patient, underlying lung disease, the severity of hypoxemia, presence of hypercapnia, and patient tolerance. The main low-flow delivery devices are nasal cannula, simple face masks, masks with a reservoir that can be either non-rebreather or partially re-breather type, and diffusor masks. The Venturi mask is a simple form of O_2 delivery system providing high flow O_2 with a relatively fixed FiO_2 making it suitable for chronic obstructive pulmonary disease (COPD) patients.

The high-flow nasal cannula has gained wide acceptance in the treatment of acute hypoxemic respiratory failure. It improves functional residual capacity and decreases work of breathing. The recommended target SpO_2 range in most patients not at risk of hypercapnic respiratory failure is 94–98% and is 88–92% in patients at risk of hypercapnic respiratory failure.

---

* Corresponding Author's Email: atopeli@hacettepe.edu.tr.

In: Nasal High Flow and Non-Invasive Ventilatory Support
Editors: A. M. Esquinas, D. A. Lagonidis, P. Silva Santos et al.
ISBN: 979-8-88697-420-1

LTOT applied by an O_2 concentrator, liquid O_2 system or compressed gas cylinder has been shown to improve survival in patients with COPD and has been recommended to be used for more than 15 hours/day. O_2 should be considered as a drug that should be prescribed and titrated at the target SpO_2 range with the appropriate method and dose by trained staff, and over-oxygenation should be avoided.

Keywords: low-flow oxygen, nasal cannula, rebreather mask, Venturi mask, high-flow oxygen, long-term oxygen, hyperbaric oxygen

Introduction

Oxygen (O_2) therapy is essential in both critically ill patients in the acute setting, and in patients with chronic respiratory failure as long-term O_2 therapy (LTOT). The main indication of O_2 therapy is the prevention and treatment of hypoxemia and tissue hypoxia. Hypoxemia denotes a low level of blood O_2, i.e., partial O_2 pressure. Hypoxia denotes low O_2 supply which is influenced by other factors such as cardiac output and hemoglobin. O_2 is not indicated for the treatment of dyspnea, nor to decrease work of breathing. Moreover, O_2 is intended to be used for oxygenation, not for the treatment of the underlying cause of respiratory failure. Work up and treatment for underlying causes of acute and chronic respiratory failure should be extensively carried out [1].

Hypoxemia: Definition and Monitoring

Hypoxemia is generally defined as partial arterial O_2 pressure (PaO_2) of less than 80 mmHg on room air, i.e., a fraction of inspired O_2 (FiO_2) 0.21 or 21%. PaO_2 less than 60 mmHg and saturation of arterial O_2 (SaO_2) less than 0.90 or 90% denote hypoxemic respiratory failure. It is more appropriate to define oxygenation by using PaO_2 to FiO_2 ratio. Normal PaO_2/FiO_2 is above 400. PaO_2/FiO_2 less than 300 is considered hypoxemic respiratory failure. In Berlin's definition of acute respiratory distress syndrome (ARDS), ARDS is classified as mild, moderate, and severe according to PaO_2/FiO_2 ratio, so that it is mild if PaO_2/FiO_2 is between 200-300, moderate if PaO_2/FiO_2 is between 100-200 and severe if PaO_2/FiO_2 is less than100 mmHg [2].

Arterial blood gas (ABG) analysis is the gold standard for diagnosis of the presence and types of respiratory failure, and to determine the severity of hypoxemia. ABG is recommended in critically-ill patients, in the presence of or worsening of hypoxemia and dyspnea, patients at risk of hypercapnic respiratory failure, patients at risk of metabolic acidosis, and patients with poor pulse oximetry signal [3]. However, due to its invasiveness, monitorization of O_2 saturation measured by a pulse oximeter (SpO_2) is the most widely used method bearing in mind its limitations in shock states, carbon monoxide (CO) poisoning, etc. Another limitation of SpO_2 is its inability to determine hyperoxia. However, SpO_2 is considered as the 5th vital sign and pulse oximetry should be widely available. Patient assessment should be performed if SpO_2 decreases more than 3% or below the target range for that patient [1].

SpO_2 cannot differentiate between carboxy- and oxy-hemoglobin so carboxy-hemoglobin should be measured through a co-oximeter in CO poisoning. PaO_2 is also normal in CO poisoning, but SaO_2 is lower in ABG and there is tissue hypoxia. Normal value of carboxy-hemoglobin in a healthy individual is less than 3%. In smokers, it might increase up to 10-15%. Levels more than 15% are pathologic [1].

As PaO_2 measurement is invasive, PaO_2/FiO_2 ratio cannot be monitored frequently and therefore SpO_2/FiO_2 could be used as a surrogate for PaO_2/FiO_2 especially in SpO_2 values less than 97%. SpO_2/FiO_2 value of 235 revealed an 85% sensitivity and specificity in predicting PaO_2/FiO_2 of 200, whereas SpO_2/FiO_2 value of 315 had 91% sensitivity and somewhat lower specificity of 56% in predicting PaO_2/FiO_2 of 300 [4].

Alveolar-arterial O_2 gradient ($P(A\text{-}a)O_2$) is another method to determine gas exchange. PAO_2 is calculated as "FiO_2 x (Patm – PH_2O) – $PaCO_2/RQ$" (Patm is atmospheric pressure which is 760 mmHg at sea level, PH_2O is the water vapor pressure of 47 cmH_2O, $PaCO_2$ is partial arterial carbon dioxide pressure and RQ is respiratory quotient which is around 0.8 under normal metabolic and diet conditions). $P(A\text{-}a)O_2$ is normally less than 15 mmHg but is dependent on age. A simplified formula of "age/4 + 4" is used to determine normal $P(A\text{-}a)O_2$ according to age. In addition, the normal value for $P(A\text{–}a)O_2$ increases with increasing FiO_2. Therefore PaO_2/FiO_2 is more frequently used in clinical practice rather than $P(A\text{–}a)O_2$ [5].

Oxygen Delivery Methods

The main O_2 source in hospitals is liquid O_2 (LOX), each liter of which provides 860 L of gaseous oxygen, making this the most efficient system for oxygen storage and transportation. Alternate sources for oxygen in the hospital setting consist of compressed gas cylinders. In addition, there are O_2 generators or large concentrators which occupy substantial physical space and can cost as much as a LOX system. However, disasters can strain these resources. Moreover, attaching many ventilators to the O_2 system may lead to the problem of depressurization, especially in old buildings. Therefore, it is important to have national, regional, and institutional master plans for disasters and not to waste O_2 [6].

O_2 is delivered from outlets in the patient areas in hospitals. It is then administered to patients through several kinds of devices attached to a flow meter. The choice of the device is determined by several factors including the clinical status of the patient, underlying lung disease if present, the severity of hypoxemia, presence of hypercapnia, and patient tolerance. Delivered FiO_2 depends on various factors such as the adjusted flow rate, delivery device, and minute ventilation of the patient.

O_2 delivery systems are generally classified as low-flow devices providing variable FiO_2 or high-flow devices providing fixed FiO_2 [1, 7, 8].

Low-Flow Delivery Devices

Low-flow devices provide O_2 at flow rates lower than patients' inspiratory demands, i.e., lower than the actual inspiratory flow of about 30 L/min. The final delivered FiO_2 depends on the ventilatory demands of the patient and the size of the oxygen reservoir. As the tidal volume and minute ventilation increase, room air is entrained and FiO_2 decreases. Therefore, FiO_2 is variable. The main low-flow delivery devices are nasal cannula, simple face masks (Hudson masks), and masks with a reservoir which can be either non-rebreather or partially re-breather type.

Nasal cannula is the most widely available and frequently used device, even for home O_2 therapy. It is convenient for the patient so that mouth is not covered allowing, eating, speaking, expectoration, etc. Although some humidification is possible, it is impaired as flow rates increase causing discomfort. Each 1 L/min increase in flow rate increases FiO_2 by about 4%. However, variable FiO_2 which is dependent on the patient's minute ventilation and extent of mouth breathing is a disadvantage. The maximum FiO_2 that could be achieved is around 45% with a flow rate of 6 L/min, above which is needless and can cause nasal dryness and patient discomfort [5]. As an example, in a patient with a tidal volume of 500 mL, respiratory frequency of

20 per minute, and inspiratory time of 1 second, receiving O_2 with nasal cannula at a flow rate of 6 L/min (100 ml/sec), there is 50 mL anatomic reservoir and 100 mL reservoir due to the nasal cannula having FiO_2 of 1.0. The remaining 350 mL tidal volume receives room air (350x0.21 = 70 mL). Therefore, FiO_2 is 220/500 = 0.44. If this patient's tidal volume decreases to 250 mL, at a flow rate of 6 L/min (100 ml/sec), there is a 50 mL anatomic reservoir and 100 mL reservoir due to the nasal cannula having FiO_2 of 1.0. The remaining 100 mL tidal volume receives room air (100x0.21 = 20 mL). Therefore, FiO_2 is 170/250 = 0.69 (9). FiO_2 increases as tidal volume and respiratory frequency decrease and vice versa.

A simple face mask can deliver about 50-60% FiO_2 at flow rates up to 10 L/min. However, FiO_2 is not precise. It might lead to CO_2 re-breathing and hypercapnia at flow rates lower than 5 L/min especially in patients with COPD.

A non-rebreather mask with a reservoir of 1000 mL can provide up to 85-95% FiO_2 at flow rates of 15 L/min. The valve between the mask and the reservoir prevents CO_2 re-breathing and the valves on the expiratory holes of the mask prevent the gas mixture from the room air. It is recommended to have a one-way valve only in one of the two exhalation ports of the face mask as a safety precaution so that the patient can still receive room air if O_2 flow is accidentally interrupted. Partially re-breather mask types do not contain these valves and FiO_2 might reach levels only up to 60-70%.

Diffusor masks (OxyMask) can deliver O_2 within a wide range of FiO_2 (24-90%) under a wide range of flow rates up to 15 L/min. It directs O_2 to the nose and mouth using a patented diffuser system. Although nose and mouth are covered, CO_2 rebreathing is not observed, and it is more comfortable than the simple mask.

For infants, a low-flow blow-by system is a convenient way of providing O_2. Hoods and tents are also suitable for infants and children.

It is important to humidify O_2, especially in flow rates > 4 L/min with a nasal cannula or FiO_2 > 35% in other systems and for prolonged periods of O_2 use to prevent the development of dry secretions and to increase patient comfort.

High-Flow Delivery Devices

These devices provide a relatively fixed amount of FiO_2 by delivering the gas at flow rates that exceed the patient's peak inspiratory flow rate and by using devices that entrain a fixed proportion of room air.

The Venturi mask was developed by the British Physician Earl James Moran Campbell based on the physical principle that when a liquid or gas flows through a narrowed tube, flow increases and pressure decreases. With the Venturi mask even if the adjusted flow rate is low, through nozzles of varying diameters and holes from where the air is entrained from outside, flow reaching the patient increases up to 50-60 L/min, providing a relatively fixed amount of FiO_2. From the nozzle providing FiO_2 of 24% at a 2 L/min flow rate, the air entrainment ratio is calculated as "(100-24)/(24-21) = 76/3 = 25.3/1". For the 2 L/min flow rate, the total flow received by the patient is (25.3x2)+2 = 52.6 L/min.

On the other hand, for the nozzle providing FiO_2 of 60% at a 15 L/min flow rate, the air entrainment ratio is "(100-60)/(60-21) = 40/39 = 1.03/1". For the 15 L/min flow rate, the total flow received by the patient is (1.03x15)+15 = 30.4 L/min. Relatively fixed FiO_2 is provided usually with nozzles of different colors. Therefore, the Venturi mask is a simple form of O_2 delivery system providing high flow O_2 with a relatively fixed FiO_2 ranging from 24-60%, making it suitable for COPD patients who should not be over-oxygenated. For patients who are breathing at a respiratory rate of more than 30/min, the flow rate is recommended to be increased [1, 10]. The FiO_2 provided by different low-flow devices and the Venturi mask according to different flow rates is shown in Table 1.

Table 1. FiO_2 provided by different low-flow devices and the Venturi mask

<table>
<tr><td></td><td colspan="6">FiO₂, %</td></tr>
<tr><td>Flow rate, L/min</td><td>Nasal cannula</td><td>Simple mask</td><td>Non-rebreather mask</td><td>Partially re-breather mask</td><td>Diffusor mask</td><td>Venturi mask</td></tr>
<tr><td>1</td><td>24</td><td></td><td></td><td></td><td>24-28</td><td></td></tr>
<tr><td>2</td><td>28</td><td></td><td></td><td></td><td>28-32</td><td>24</td></tr>
<tr><td>3</td><td>32</td><td></td><td></td><td></td><td>30-60</td><td></td></tr>
<tr><td>4</td><td>36</td><td></td><td></td><td></td><td rowspan="3">35-70</td><td>28</td></tr>
<tr><td>5</td><td>40</td><td>40</td><td></td><td></td><td></td></tr>
<tr><td>6</td><td>44</td><td>40-50</td><td></td><td></td><td>31</td></tr>
<tr><td>7</td><td></td><td>50-60</td><td></td><td></td><td rowspan="3">50-80</td><td></td></tr>
<tr><td>8</td><td></td><td rowspan="8">60</td><td></td><td></td><td>35</td></tr>
<tr><td>9</td><td></td><td></td><td></td><td></td></tr>
<tr><td>10</td><td></td><td rowspan="6">>85</td><td rowspan="6">60-70</td><td rowspan="6">60-90</td><td>40</td></tr>
<tr><td>11</td><td></td><td></td></tr>
<tr><td>12</td><td></td><td></td></tr>
<tr><td>13</td><td></td><td></td></tr>
<tr><td>14</td><td></td><td></td></tr>
<tr><td>15</td><td></td><td>60</td></tr>
</table>

High-flow nasal cannula (HFNC) is being used widely as it has several advantages and is simple to use. Early initiation is recommended to avoid non-invasive and invasive mechanical ventilation and to avoid re-intubation after extubation. HFNC is superior to non-invasive ventilation in acute hypoxemic respiratory failure. It consists of a flow generator, active heated humidifier, single heated circuit, and nasal cannula. The heated humidified oxygen is delivered through a wide-bore nasal prong at flow rates up to 60 L/min and FiO_2 up to 100%.

This flow improves functional residual capacity by providing some positive end-expiratory pressure (PEEP) if the mouth is closed, and humidification enhances mucociliary clearance of secretions, both effects leading to a reduction in the work of breathing. In addition, it does not increase dead space ventilation and is comfortable for the patient. Nasopharyngeal washout and PEEP increase tidal volume, decrease respiratory rate, and reduce auto-PEEP. Thoraco-abdominal synchronization is improved with HFNC. Even with mouth breathing, FiO_2 is preserved due to the anatomic reservoir, however, PEEP decreases with mouth breathing [11, 12].

Oxygen Administration

SpO_2 target of 94-96% is appropriate for most critically ill patients [13]. However, guidelines recommend a SpO_2 range of 94-98% [1, 3, 12]. The exceptions are patients with CO poisoning, air embolism, sickle cell crisis, cluster-type headache, and pneumothorax. In addition, in hypercapnic patients or for those at risk of hypercapnia the target SpO_2 should even be lower, i.e., 88-92%.

In severely hypoxemic critically-ill patients, oxygenation could be started with a non-rebreather mask with a reservoir at a 15 L/min flow rate aiming for SpO_2 of 94-98% even if the patient is at risk of hypercapnic respiratory failure pending ABG results. Other low-flow devices and the Venturi mask are also appropriate if SpO_2 is at the target level. Once the patient is stable, FiO_2 is reduced aiming at the target SpO_2. HFNC is appropriate if high FiO_2 is required for a prolonged period.

In hypoxemic patients with a serious illness requiring moderate amounts of oxygen, oxygenation could be started with nasal cannula at flow rates of 2-6 L/min, a simple facemask at flow rates of 5-10 L/min, or other devices aiming for a SpO_2 target of 94–98%. If SpO_2 cannot be maintained or initial SpO_2 is less than 85%, a non-rebreather mask with a reservoir at a 15 L/min flow rate could be used. If there is a risk of hypercapnic respiratory failure SpO_2 target would be 88-92%. If ABG shows normal $PaCO_2$, SpO_2 target could be increased up to 94-98%. ABG is recommended to be repeated after 30-60 minutes. However, if the patient has a history of previous hypercapnic respiratory failure, a history of non-invasive or invasive ventilation, is older than 50 years of age with a long-term smoking history and dyspnea then the patient could be presumed as COPD, and the target SpO_2 should remain at 88–92%.

In a patient with COPD or other conditions at risk of hypercapnic respiratory failure who requires low dose O_2, it is appropriate to start with a Venturi mask at a FiO_2 of 24% or a nasal cannula of 1-2 L/min, aiming for a SpO_2 of 88–92%. If the patient is hypercapnic and acidotic, despite 30 minutes of appropriate treatment and oxygenation, non-invasive ventilation should be considered [1, 3]. O_2 should be weaned as long as the patient is stable and is on 1-2 L/min low-flow O_2 [1].

Adverse Effects of Oxygen Treatment

O_2 toxicity in the lungs is a concern with FiO_2 at more than 60%. It is believed to result from the formation of excessive reactive oxygen species. Acute tracheobronchitis is the earliest clinical syndrome that can occur within a few hours. Prolonged exposures may induce diffuse alveolar damage with similar clinical findings as ARDS which might finally lead to pulmonary fibrosis.

In a systematic review including studies on patients with sepsis, critical illness, stroke, trauma, acute myocardial infarction (AMI), or cardiac arrest, and patients who had emergency surgery, liberal O_2 therapy as compared to conservative O_2 therapy was associated with increased in-hospital mortality. Thus, supplemental oxygen targeting SpO_2 of more than 94-96% might be unfavorable and it is recommended to stop supplemental O_2 if SpO_2 is more than 96% [13].

For patients with AMI or stroke, it is strongly recommended not to initiate O_2 therapy if SpO_2 is equal to or more than 93% and weakly recommended not to initiate O_2 therapy if SpO_2 is 90-92%. It is suggested to aim SpO_2 <96% under supplemental O_2. In patients with stroke and SpO_2 of 90-92%, hospital mortality was reported to be higher in patients who received supplemental O_2 compared to patients who did not receive O_2. In patients with AMI, coronary revascularisation within 6 months and recurrent AMI up to 1 year were reported to be higher in patients who received supplemental O_2 compared to patients who did not receive O_2 [14].

Over-oxygenation might exacerbate hypercapnia in chronically hypercapnic patients such as COPD mainly due to worsening of ventilation-perfusion (V/Q) matching by impairing hypoxic pulmonary vasoconstriction which normally improves V/Q matching. Therefore, over-oxygenation might increase dead space ventilation. The other mechanism is the Haldane effect which is the rightward displacement of the carbon dioxide (CO_2)-hemoglobin dissociation curve in the presence of increased oxygen saturation. Supplemental O_2 displaces CO_2 from hemoglobin increasing the amount of dissolved CO_2. And finally, supplemental O_2 blunts hypoxemic drive which has a minor contribution to hypercapnia. Nevertheless, even in hypercapnic patients, the primary aim is to correct hypoxemia [5].

Long-Term Oxygen Therapy

LTOT is indicated when PaO_2 is equal to or less than 55 mmHg at rest, during exercise, or at sleep, and in patients with PaO_2 less than 60 mmHg, if cor pulmonale is present. LTOT has been shown to improve survival in patients with COPD and has been recommended to be used for more than 15 hours/day. The best way to deliver LTOT is with an O_2 concentrator, also called an O_2 generator, which can be stationary or portable. For most patients, stationary concentrators are convenient. Portable ones are recommended for people who use LTOT outside the home. An O_2 concentrator draws room air which is filtered and nitrogen is absorbed, and then drawn out to the atmosphere, leaving concentrated oxygen (90% or higher). Most concentrators deliver O_2 at flow rates up to 5 L/min, with some concentrators delivering flow rates up to 10 L/min. O_2 can be delivered by either continuous flow or in pulse mode. Continuous flow delivery supplies a constant, steady, and reliable O_2 flow while pulse mode delivers a pulsed bolus of O_2 during inspiration. The main advantage of O_2 concentrators is that they run on electrical power and do not need to be refilled, which can be a disadvantage if there is a power cut, thus a backup is needed.

A compressed gas cylinder could be used as a backup system for a concentrator at home and as a temporary oxygen supply system during transport of the O_2 or ventilator-dependent patient. A cylinder is a metal container filled with compressed gas under high pressure. They are available in different sizes with different O_2 capacities. They can be portable cylinders, lightweight cylinders, or home-fill cylinders. They are colored white to distinguish them from other gases. A regulator is attached to the cylinder's top for adjustment of O_2 flow. The capacity of cylinders is quite limited as such a 400 L cylinder under 200 bar pressure can last 2.5 hours at a low-flow rate. Home-fill cylinders can be refilled by an oxygen concentrator. O_2-conserving devices can be used to deliver pulse-mode O_2 and can reduce O_2 usage by 50%. They enable cylinders to last longer and reduce cost. However, SpO_2 may not be stable and patients with advanced chronic lung disease might not be able to trigger the conserving device at inspiration efficiently.

LOX system can also be used for domiciliary O_2 LTOT. It spares space as each liter of liquid O_2 releases 860 L of gaseous O_2. LOX which has a minimum of 99.5% purity must first be vaporized into a compressed gas and then warmed at the ambient temperature inside the equipment before the patient receives O_2. There is a larger stationary LOX system inside homes, with smaller portable systems that can be refilled and used outside the home. For ambulatory patients, the LOX system can be more convenient and safer than cylinders because they are under lower pressure. The portable LOX systems last longer than other portable systems and are relatively lighter. The main disadvantage of LOX systems is that they require a larger home LOX system which has to be filled regularly and this might increase the cost.

Patients eligible for LTOT should be initiated on a flow rate of 1 L/min and titrated up in 1 L/min increment until SpO_2 is more than >90%. Non-hypercapnic patients should increase their flow rate by 1 L/min during sleep in the absence of any contraindications. There is no need for humidification in LTOT under low flow rates and unless the patient has a tracheostomy [8, 9, 15, 16].

Hyperbaric Oxygen Therapy

O_2 can also be administered at pressures higher than 1 atm, named hyperbaric O_2 (HBO). It can be applied in a small single-patient chamber or a large multi-place chamber. The chamber is filled with compressed air while the patients breathe 100% O_2 through masks or hoods.

Under 1 atm pressure (760 mmHg at sea level) and on room air (FiO_2 21%), PAO_2 would be around 104 mmHg, with a respiratory quotient of 0.8. Under normobaric conditions and 100% FiO_2, PAO_2 would be around 670 mmHg. However, under 3 atm HBO and 100% FiO_2, PAO_2 would be around 2200 mmHg increasing the dissolved O_2. An increase in dissolved O_2 causes an increase in O_2 diffusion to the tissues. The main indications of HBO are air embolism and CO poisoning where hemoglobin's oxygen-carrying capacity has been impaired. Central nervous system toxicity such as generalized or focal convulsions is a major concern during HBO treatment. Dizziness, blurred vision, tinnitus, hypercapnia, and barotrauma to the ears, sinuses, and lungs are other side effects. Therefore, the sessions are usually held for less than 2 hours under less than 2.8 atm pressure [17].

Conclusion

We consider that:

- O_2 is the most widely used medical gas, and
- O_2 is indicated to treat hypoxemia, not breathlessness, and not the underlying cause of respiratory failure.

It is like a drug that should be prescribed and titrated at the target saturation range with the appropriate method and dose by trained staff. The recommended oxygen target saturation range in patients not at risk of hypercapnic respiratory failure is 94–98% and in patients at risk of hypercapnic respiratory failure is 88–92%. In most acutely ill patients, over-oxygenation should be avoided.

References

[1] O'Driscoll BR, Howard LS, Earis J, Vak M on behalf of the British Thoracic Society Emergency Oxygen Guideline Group. BTS guideline for oxygen use in adults in healthcare and emergency settings. *Thorax* 2017; 72: i1–i90.

[2] ARDS Definition Task Force: Ranieri VM, Rubenfeld GD, Thompson BT, Ferguson ND, Caldwell E, Fan E, Camporota L, Slutsky AS, Antonelli M, Anzueto A, Beale R, Brochard L, Brower R, Esteban A, Gattinoni L, Rhodes A, Vincent JL, Bersten A, Needham D, Pesenti A. Acute respiratory distress syndrome: the Berlin definition. *JAMA* 2012; 307: 2526-33.

[3] Kane B, Decalmer S, O'Driscoll BR. Emergency oxygen therapy: from guideline to implementation. *Breathe* 2013; 9: 247-54.

[4] Rice TW, Wheeler A, Bernard G, Hayden DL, Schoenfeld DA, Ware LB, for the NIH, NHLBI ARDS Network. Comparison of the SpO_2/FIO_2 ratio and the PaO_2/FIO_2 ratio in patients with acute lung injury or ARDS. *Chest* 2007; 132: 410-7.

[5] Petersson J, Glenny RW. Gas exchange and ventilation–perfusion relationships in the lung. *Eur Resp J* 2014; 44: 1023-41.
[6] Blakeman TC, Branson RD. Oxygen supplies in disaster management. *Resp Care* 2013; 58: 173–82.
[7] Ortac Ersoy E, Topeli A. Oxygen therapy systems in respiratory failure (Turkish). *Yogun Bakim Derg* (current name *J Crit Intensive Care*) 2016; 7: 99-105.
[8] Hardavella G, Karampinis I, Frille A, Sreter K, Rousalova I. Oxygen devices and delivery systems. *Breathe* 2019; 15: e108–e16.
[9] McCoy RW. Options for Home Oxygen Therapy Equipment: Storage and Metering of Oxygen in the Home. *Resp Care* 2013; 58: 65-85.
[10] Soto-Ruiz KM, Peacock F, Varon J. The men and history behind the venturi mask. *Resuscitation* 2011; 82: 244–6.
[11] Nishimura M. High-flow nasal cannula oxygen therapy devices. *Respir Care* 2019; 64: 735–42.
[12] Piraino T, Madden M, Roberts KJ, Lamberti J, Ginier E, Strickland SL. AARC clinical practice guideline: management of adult patients with oxygen in the acute care setting. *Respir Care* 2022; 67: 115–128.
[13] Chu DK, Kim LHY, Young PJ, Zamiri N, Almenawer SA, Jaeschke R, Szczeklik W, Schünemann HJ, Neary JD, Alhazzani W. Mortality and morbidity in acutely ill adults treated with liberal versus conservative oxygen therapy (IOTA):a systematic review and meta-analysis. *Lancet* 2018; 391: 1693–705.
[14] Siemieniuk RAC, Chu DK, Kim LHY, Güell-Rous MR, Alhazzani W, Soccal PM, Karanicolas PJ, Farhoumand PD, Siemieniuk JLK, Satia I, Irusen EM, Refaat MM, Mikita JS, Smith M, Cohen DN, Vandvik PO, Agoritsas T, Lytvyn L, Guyatt GH. Oxygen therapy for acutely ill medical patients: a clinical practice guideline. *BMJ* 2018; 363: k4169.
[15] Hardinge M, Annandale J, Bourne S, Cooper B, Evans A, Freeman D, Green A, Hippolyte S, Knowles V, MacNee W, McDonnell L, Pye K, Suntharalingam J, Vora V, Wilkinson T, British Thoracic Society Home Oxygen Guideline Development Group, on behalf of the British Thoracic Society Standards of Care Committee. British Thoracic Society guidelines for home oxygen use in adults. *Thorax* 2015; 70: i1-i43.
[16] Jacobs SS, Krishnan JA, Lederer DJ, Ghazipura M, Hossain T, Tan AYM, Carlin B, Drummond MB, Ekstrom M, Garvey C, Graney BA, Jackson B, Kallstrom T, Knight SL, Lindell K, Prieto-Centurion V, Renzoni EA, Ryerson CJ, Schneidman A, Swigris J, Upson D, Holland AE; on behalf of the American Thoracic Society Assembly on Nursing. Home oxygen therapy for adults with chronic lung disease: an official American Thoracic Society clinical practice guideline. *Am J Respir Crit Care Med* 2020; 202: e121–41.
[17] Bitterman H. Bench-to-bedside review: Oxygen as a drug. *Crit Care* 2009; 13: 205.

Chapter 2

Physiology

Alexander J. Sweidan, MD
Luqman Nasouf, MD
and Catherine S. H. Sassoon*, **MD**
Division of Pulmonary and Critical Care Medicine,
Department of Medicine, University of California, Irvine, California, USA

Abstract

In this chapter, we review the primary evidence for the six known physiologic effects of high-flow nasal cannula oxygen therapy in the adults, and examine:

1) The use of high-flow nasal cannula to deliver a precise fraction of inspired oxygen (FIO_2) when the flow rate exceeds the patients' peak inspiratory flow rate;
2) The dependence of upper airway expiratory resistance on the size of the nasal cannula prongs;
3) The ability of high-flow nasal cannula oxygen therapy to prevent rebreathing of carbon dioxide by washing it out of anatomic dead space, thus promoting inspiration of oxygen;
4) The ability of high-flow nasal cannula oxygen therapy to improve breathing patterns dependent on states of wakefulness and sleep, specifically by reducing respiratory rate during wakefulness;
5) The ability of high-flow nasal cannula oxygen therapy to induce positive airway pressure and positive end-expiratory pressure;

* Corresponding Author's Email: csassoon@uci.edu.

In: Nasal High Flow and Non-Invasive Ventilatory Support
Editors: A. M. Esquinas, D. A. Lagonidis, P. Silva Santos et al.
ISBN: 979-8-88697-420-1

6) The use of high-flow nasal cannula oxygen therapy to reduce pressure-time product or metabolic work of breathing.

We also examine the plausible adverse effects of oxygen toxicity as a direct result of high-flow nasal cannula oxygen therapy when the set FIO_2 remains high for a prolonged duration.

Keywords: upper airway expiratory resistance, anatomic dead space, positive airway pressure, positive end-expiratory pressure, metabolic work of breathing

Introduction

In the last two decades, high-flow nasal cannula (HFNC) oxygen (O_2) therapy has been the mainstay of non-invasive modality in the pediatric intensive care unit (ICU). The therapy also has become part of the non-invasive therapeutic armamentarium in the adult ICU, especially because it reduces 90-day mortality compared with non-invasive ventilation or conventional oxygen therapy [1]. Currently HFNC also has been employed in non-ICU areas and domiciliary use for patients with chronic obstructive pulmonary disease (COPD) [2].

High-flow nasal cannula O_2 therapy consists of the delivery of heated, humidified, high-flow O_2 via a heated single-limb circuit and nasal cannula with a precisely set flow rate and inspired oxygen fraction (FIO_2). The range and maximum flow rate depend on the patient population: In pediatrics, flow rates range from 1 L/min/Kg body weight to a maximum of 10 to 12 L/min [3]. In adults, flow rates can be set to a maximum of 40 or 60 L/min, depending on the manufacturer of the HFNC [4]. The oxygen-air blender allows the FIO_2 to be set between 21% and 100%. The set flow rate is of paramount importance for achieving the beneficial effects of HFNC.

The objective of this chapter is to review the following physiologic effects of HFNC O_2 therapy in adults:

1) FIO_2 approximates or equals the delivered O_2 concentration;
2) Increased upper airway resistance;
3) Clearance of carbon dioxide (CO_2) from anatomic dead space;
4) Improved breathing patterns;
5) Development of positive airway pressure and positive end-expiratory pressure (PEEP);

6) Reduced pressure-time product and metabolic work of breathing.

Physiological Effects of HFNC

Actual FIO_2 Approximates or Equals the Delivered O_2 Concentration

With conventional O_2 delivery, flow rate is commonly limited to 15 L/min. Because the peak flow rate of patients with acute respiratory failure can be extremely high (120 L/min or greater), excessive entrainment of room air results in the variability of FIO_2 [4]. The use of HFNC circumvents the FIO_2 variability because the delivered flow rate can be set higher than the patient's peak inspiratory flow (PIF) rate. In a study of healthy subjects breathing at rest with mouth open or closed, an O_2 concentration of 60% was administered via HFNC with the flow rates varied randomly at 10, 20, 30, 40, and 50 L/min [5]. Expired O_2 (FEO_2) and expired CO_2 ($FECO_2$) concentrations were measured using oxygraphy and capnography, respectively, via a catheter inserted in the hypopharynx. FIO_2 was calculated from FEO_2 and $FECO_2$ using the alveolar gas equation, assuming FEO_2 equals to alveolar O_2 fraction. The average PIF rate at rest was 28 L/min. At flow rates above 30 L/min with closed-mouth breathing, FIO_2 approached the set O_2 concentration of 60% but was lower with mouth open. During exercise, average PIF rate was 120 L/min. At a set flow rate of 50 L/min, the average calculated FIO_2 was 35%, lower than the set O_2 concentration of 60%. This study demonstrated the importance of HFNC set flow rate in delivering the desired or actual FIO_2; however, a similar study has not been performed in critically ill patients.

In a bench study using lung simulation with a nasal cavity model connected to the HFNC, Sun et al. (6) sought the variables affecting delivered or actual FIO_2. They tested various combinations of HFNC set flow rates of 20, 40, 60, and 80 L/min and set O_2 concentrations of 30%, 50%, and 70%. The simulated lung PIF rate was set at 40, 80, or 120 L/min, tidal volume (VT) at 400 or 600 ml, and respiratory rate (RR) at 20/min. Using regression analysis, the calculated actual FIO_2 delivered is as follows:

$$\text{Actual } FIO_2 = (0.78 \times \text{set-}FIO_2) + (0.17 \times \text{set-flow}) - (0.09 \times \text{PIF}) + 2.71$$

This equation, however, has not been prospectively validated in clinical study.

In summary, to achieve the desired or actual FIO_2, it is essential for the HFNC set flow rate to exceed the patient's PIF rate.

Increased Expiratory Upper Airway Resistance as Function of the Nasal Cannula Size

A high-flow nasal cannula delivers the flow of O_2 through the patient's nostrils, generally with mouth closed. The set flow rate and the size of the cannula influence the upper airway resistance. Recently, using a 3D-printed human upper airway model, Adams et al. (7) measured upper airway resistance with varying set flow rates and nasal cannulas of small, medium, and large sizes, and then calculated the resistive work of breathing using data (respiratory rate (RR), minute volume, Inspiratory: Expiratory (I:E) ratio) from published studies on humans receiving HFNC. The large nasal cannula produces greater expiratory resistance than the small cannula. With a set flow rate of 40 L/min and tracheal flow of 30 L/min, the expiratory upper airway resistance via the large cannula was 20% higher than that of the small cannula. With the large nasal cannula, the leak area between the cannula prong and the nostril contributes to the rise in pressure as the exhaled flow passes through the narrower area, resulting in greater pressure loss. Despite the increase in expiratory upper airway resistance, the total resistive work of breathing (Joules/min) required to produce tracheal flow through the upper airway is reduced through a drop in inspiratory resistive work when RR and minute volume decrease with HFNC treatment.

In summary, the degree of upper airway expiratory resistance is proportional to the size of the nasal cannula, whereas the total resistive work of breathing to overcome the resistance is reduced only when the HFNC set flow rate results in reduced RR and minute volume.

Clearance of CO_2 from Anatomic Dead Space

Möller et al. [8] demonstrated the efficacy of HFNC to clear CO_2 from anatomic dead space and prevent rebreathing of CO_2. The investigators studied CO_2 clearance in healthy nonsmoking subjects, using 81m Krypton (81mKr) gas scintigraphy during a closed-mouth breath-holding maneuver. With an HFNC set flow rate of 15, 30, and 45 L/min and CO_2 clearance as a function of the HFNC set flow rate, the average clearance rates were 41, 53, and 73 ml/s, respectively. Fast clearance occurred in the anterior and posterior nasal cavity and were longer beyond the soft palate. At a HFNC flow rate of 45 L/min, the average clearance half-lives ($T_{1/2}$) of 81mKr in the anterior and posterior nasal cavities, pharynx, and trachea were 0.4, 0.5, 4.4, and 10.5 seconds, respectively.

In the same study, the use of HFNC to prevent patients from rebreathing CO_2 was evaluated in tracheostomized subjects who had been weaned from mechanical ventilation. The tracheostomy tube was replaced with a tracheostomy retainer, from which CO_2 and O_2 concentrations were measured with CO_2 and O_2 gas analyzers, respectively, and inspired volume was estimated by means of respiratory inductance plethysmography. With the first inspired volume of 100 mL and a HFNC set flow rate of 45 L/min, the inspired concentration of CO_2 was the lowest, whereas inspired O_2 concentration was the highest. A decrease in inspired CO_2 concentration (approximately 0%) was associated with an increase (approximately 21%) in O_2 concentration as a function of the HFNC set flow rates.

In summary, HFNC clears the upper airways of $FECO_2$, which reduces anatomic dead space, lessens the amount of CO_2 that is rebreathed in a manner dependent on flow rate, and increases O_2 in the inspired gas, making ventilation more efficient.

Improved Breathing Patterns Influenced by States of Wakefulness and Sleep

A high-flow nasal cannula improves breathing patterns that are influenced by the states of wakefulness and sleep. Mündel et al. (9] examined the breathing patterns during wakefulness and sleep states in ten healthy subjects, with and without HFNC at set flow rates of 15, 30, and 45 L/min. Values for VT and RR were measured using respiratory inductive plethysmography. During wakefulness with HFNC, RR decreased, whereas VT increased with preserved minute ventilation. The decrease in RR is a function of HFNC set flow rates and is due to prolonged expiratory time compared to breathing without HFNC (average 6.0 s expiratory time with HFNC at 45 L/min versus 3.1 s expiratory time in the control without HFNC).

The mechanisms of reduced RR during wakefulness remain unclear. Similar to the study of Adams et al. [7], Mündel et al. [9] using a nasal cavity model, demonstrated that HFNC decreased upper airway inspiratory resistance and induced small positive airway pressure during inhalation.

Depending on the size of the cannula, upper airway expiratory resistance increased with higher peak expiratory flow rate during exhalation, producing positive end expiratory airway pressure. Taken together, those factors may contribute to the reduced RR during wakefulness.

In contrast to the wakefulness state, during sleep, RR remained constant, VT decreased, and, consequently, minute ventilation diminished. The mechanisms of reduced minute ventilation with HFNC during sleep remain unclear, however. The reduced inspiratory upper airway resistance may be associated with reduced respiratory drive, and both CO_2 clearance from the anatomical dead space and reduced CO_2 production may account for the decreased minute ventilation.

The decrease in RR with HFNC also was demonstrated in critically ill patients with acute hypoxemic respiratory failure associated with increased regional lung volume that was estimated using electrical impedance tomography [10]. However, unlike with healthy subjects, VT did not change. The reduced RR and increased regional lung volume despite unchanged VT improves lung strain, inhomogeneity, and gas exchange. Similar to patients with acute hypoxemic respiratory failure, patients with acute hypercapnic respiratory failure who received HFNC O_2 therapy post-extubation also demonstrated reduced RR with unchanged VT when compared to those receiving non-invasive ventilation.

In summary, breathing pattern responses with HFNC are affected by wakefulness and sleep states, with decreased RR during wakefulness in both healthy and critically ill subjects, although VT responses differ between groups. During sleep, RR does not change, but VT decreases. This suggests that in both wakefulness and sleep, HFNC may be beneficial in decreasing respiratory load despite different responses in RR and VT.

Development of Positive Airway Pressure and PEEP

As demonstrated in in vitro studies using a nasal cavity model, HFNC produced little positive airway pressure at the end of inhalation relative to the set flow rate: 0.5 cm H_2O at a flow rate of 15 L/min [9] and 1.5 cm H_2O at 60 L/min [7]. In a prospective study of healthy subjects (n = 15), in which airway pressure was measured via a 10 French catheter inserted into the nasopharynx and connected to a pressure transducer, Parke et al.[11] evaluated the effect of close-mouthed HFNC on mean airway pressure, changes in end-expiratory lung volume, and RR. A specially constructed HFNC system capable of delivering a maximum flow rate of 100 L/min was used. Changes in end-expiratory lung volume were estimated using electrical impedance tomography. Measurements were made at baseline of 0 flow, at set flow rates of 30 L/min to 100 L/min, in increments of 10 L/min for 1 min each augmented flow, and at washout over a period of 5 min. The mean airway pressure was a function of HFNC set flow rates with an increment of 1.2 cm H_2O per 10 L/min of increase in flow. At 100 L/min, 60 L/min, and 40 L/min, the average mean airway pressure was 11.9 cm H_2O (range, 7.2-16.2 cm H_2O); 6.1 cm H_2O (range, 4.2-8.6 cm H_2O) and 3.8 cm H_2O (range, 2.6-5.4 cm H_2O), respectively. The investigators demonstrated a linear relationship between the increase in end-expiratory lung volume and the reduced RR with increasing HFNC set flow rates. The latter observation was consistent with that of Mündel et al., [9] in awake subjects.

In addition to mean airway pressure, HFNC also induces PEEP. In the previously mentioned bench study, Sun et al. [6] evaluated the variables affecting PEEP generation with HFNC, using lung simulation with a nasal cavity model. Using multivariate regression analysis, the researchers found that the HFNC set flow rates, PIF, and VT all affected PEEP with the set flow rate as the major determinant, according to the following equation:

$$\text{PEEP} = (0.15 \times \text{set-flow}) - (0.02 \times \text{PIF}) + (0.01 \times \text{VT}) + 1.35$$

As with the determinants of FIO_2 [6], the equation has not been validated in clinical study in healthy or critically ill subjects.

In another study of ten healthy subjects (5 male and five female), Groves and Tobin [12] measured end-expiratory pressure via a 10 French catheter, inserted through the nose to the oropharynx, with HFNC flow rates set from 0 to 60 L/min on room air with mouth closed and open. End-expiratory pharyngeal pressure (EPP), a surrogate for PEEP, increased in a linear fashion by 0.8 cm H_2O per 10 L/min of increase in flow. With mouth closed, a set flow rate of 40 L/min yielded an average EPP of 5.5 cm H_2O, and at 60 L/min, the average EPP was 7.4 cm H_2O. Unfortunately, an open mouth results in a significant loss of pressure: under this condition, EPP was 2.2 cm H_2O at a flow rate of 40 L/min and 2.7 cm H_2O at a flow rate of 60 L/min.

In summary, HFNC generates positive airway pressure and end-expiratory airway pressure associated with increased end-expiratory lung volumes that are largely dependent on the magnitude of the HFNC set flow rates with the mouth closed. Improvement in end-expiratory lung volume was not influenced by body position [13].

Reduced Pressure-Time Product and Metabolic Work of Breathing

As discussed above, HFNC has several beneficial effects that are relevant to the metabolic work of breathing. Examination of the reduced upper airway inspiratory resistance, CO_2 clearance from anatomical dead space and prevention of CO_2 rebreathing, reduced RR, positive airway pressure, and PEEP generation with ensuing augmented end-expiratory lung volume elucidate the reduced inspiratory metabolic work of breathing. However, the mechanisms of the reduced metabolic work of breathing may not be attributed to the previously cited factors; variability exists, particularly in terms of breathing patterns. Studies comparing HFNC with non-invasive ventilation in patients with acute exacerbation of COPD did not show inferiority of HFNC. The reduced metabolic work with HFNC has been demonstrated in patients with acute hypoxemic respiratory failure [10] as well as in patients with hypercapnic respiratory failure following extubation from invasive mechanical ventilation [13].

Mauri et al. [10] measured the esophageal pressure-time product in fifteen patients with acute hypoxemic respiratory failure, using the patients as their own control. Measurements were taken while the patients breathed with a conventional face mask on at a flow rate of 12 L/min and then with HFNC at a flow rate of 40 L/min, in random order for 20 min each. The FIO_2 was adjusted by the attending physician to achieve oxygen saturation, which was estimated using pulse oximetry (SpO_2) of 90% to 95% with a final FIO_2 of 60% for both arms. With HFNC, changes in esophageal pressure (DPes), a measure of inspiratory effort, decreased significantly by 19%. Measures of inspiratory metabolic work of breathing, esophageal pressure-time product per breath (PTP, cm $H_2O \cdot s$) and PTP per minute (PTP × RR, cm $H_2O \cdot s/min$), also decreased significantly by 22% and 28%, respectively. Similarly, RR decreased significantly by 8%.

Di Mussi et al. [14] studied the effects of HFNC on the metabolic work of the diaphragm in 14 COPD patients extubated from invasive mechanical ventilation (Servo-i ventilator; Maquet, Getinge Group, Maquet Critical Care AB, Solna, Sweden) for acute hypercapnic respiratory failure. Patients received conventional oxygen therapy by means of a face mask with flow set at 10 L/min, interposed between two periods of HFNC for 30 min each. The HFNC flow rate was initially set at 20 L/min and was increased by 5 to 10 L/min to comfort, to a maximum of 60 L/min. The FIO_2 was titrated to the target SpO_2 of 88% to 92%. Diaphragmatic electrical activity (EAdi) was measured with a special EAdi catheter, and the signal was analyzed using the ventilator-equipped software. Neuroventilatory drive was estimated from the peak ($EAdi_{PEAK}$) and slope ($EAdi_{SLOPE}$) of EAdi. The metabolic work of breathing of the diaphragm was estimated from the inspiratory transdiaphragmatic pressure-time product per breath (PTPdi/b) and the inspiratory transdiaphragmatic pressure-time product per minute (PTPdi/min). Transdiaphragmatic pressure (Pdi) was derived from neuromechanical efficiency (NME) of the diaphragm. Using end-expiratory occlusion during 5 to 10 s, the ratio of negative airway opening pressure (P_{AW}) generated against the occlusion to EAdiPEAK is the diaphragm's neuromuscular efficiency.

Under the static condition $\Delta P_{AW} = \Delta P_{ES}$, the NME can be used to convert EAdi to Pdi, in which Pdi = NME × EAdi. Hence, PTPdi/b and PTPdi/min can be calculated. Table 1 shows the FIO_2, arterial blood gases, RR, neuroventilatory drive, and diaphragmatic metabolic work of breathing with HFNC and conventional O_2 breathing. When patients were on HFNC, FIO_2 was 46%, compared with 80% when they were on conventional O_2. Arterial PCO_2 and RR on HFNC were similar to those resulting from conventional O_2 breathing. Neuroventilatory drive and diaphragmatic metabolic work were significantly reduced with HFNC compared with conventional O_2. Five of the fourteen patients required reintubation, which reflects the severity of the underlying lung disease because all patients had undergone a similar protocol for this study.

Table 1. Gas exchange, breathing pattern, neuroventilatory drive and diaphragmatic metabolic work of breathing during period of conventional oxygen therapy interposed between periods of high flow nasal cannula

	HFNC1	*Conventional O_2*	*HFNC2*
Applied FIO_2	0.46 ± 0.10*	0.80 ± 0.19	0.46 ± 0.12*
pH	7.45 ± 0.07	7.44 ± 0.08	7.46 ± 0.08
$PaCO_2$ (mm Hg)	49.9 ± 11.9	51.8 ± 12.7	50.1 ± 12.6
PaO_2 (mm Hg)	75.1 ± 6.9	72.9 ± 8.6	81.2 ± 8.0
Respiratory Rate (breaths/min)	20.5 ± 2.9	21.4 ± 4.0	20.0 ± 1.9
TI_{NEUR} (s)	0.92 ± 0.21	0.95 ± 0.22	0.92 ± 0.17
$EAdi_{PEAK}$ (mV)	15.4 ± 6.4*	23.6 ± 10.5	15.2 ± 6.4*
$EAdi_{SLOPE}$ (mV/s)	18.6 ± 6.5*	24.0 ± 14.7	17.6 ± 10.2*
PTPdi/b (cm H2O·s)	6.7 ± 2.7*	9.9 ± 3.1	6.7 ± 2.8*
PTPdi/min (cm H2O·s/min)	135 ± 60*	211 ± 70	132 ± 56*

Values are mean ± SD. *$P < 0.05$ compared to conventional on face mask O_2 breathing (ANOVA with Bonferroni correction). Definition of abbreviations:

- HFNC1 and HFNC2: high flow nasal cannula first and second periods,
- FIO_2: inspired oxygen fraction
- $PaCO_2$: partial pressure of arterial carbon dioxide
- PaO_2: partial pressure of arterial oxygen
- TI_{NEUR}: neural inspiratory time
- $EAdi_{PEAK}$: peak diaphragm electrical activity
- $EAdi_{SLOPE}$: slope from onset to peak of diaphragm electrical activity
- PTPdi/b: inspiratory transdiaphragmatic pressure-time product per breath
- PTPdi/min: inspiratory transdiaphragmatic pressure-time product per minute (Adapted from Di Mussi et al., [14].

In summary, HFNC reduced the metabolic work of breathing in patients with both hypoxemic and hypercapnic respiratory failure; however, the breathing pattern responses differed: RR decreased in hypoxemic respiratory failure and remained unchanged in hypercapnic respiratory failure.

Oxygen Toxicity as a Plausible Adverse Effect of HFNC

The precise delivery of O_2 concentration is one of the known beneficial effects of HFNC. When the HFNC set flow rate exceeds the patient's PIF, the patient receives the actual set FIO_2. When HFNC is the initial non-invasive treatment of patients with acute hypoxemic respiratory failure, the FIO_2 with HFNC may be set at 100% to achieve SpO_2 between 92% and 96%. Although it is currently not possible to measure the FIO_2 at the alveolar level, one can assume that the exposure is close to 100% FIO_2.

With the recent Coronavirus disease (COVID-19) pandemic, patients with severe acute respiratory syndrome due to coronavirus-2 (SARS-CoV-2) may receive HFNC at FIO_2 of 100% for over 3-5 days because most of these patients are not dyspneic or demonstrated increased work of breathing for impending intubation. The benefits of oxygen for cellular respiration are clear, but there are deleterious effects because of high concentrations of FIO_2 and systemic oxygenation [15]. To our knowledge, the contribution of HFNC O_2 therapy to fatal oxygen toxicity in patients with SARS-CoV2 because of lengthy treatment with high FIO_2 has not been systematically evaluated.

Conclusion

There are several beneficial physiologic effects of HFNC, and understanding these effects allows physicians to apply this modality as the initial non-invasive treatment in both acute hypoxemic and hypercapnic respiratory failure. The beneficial effect of HFNC is a function of the set flow rate. However, the plausible adverse effects of oxygen toxicity with HFNC when 100% FIO_2 is used with high flow rate for extended periods of time is unclear and needs further study.

References

[1] Frat J P, Thille A W, Mercat A, Girault C, Ragot S, Perbet S, Prat G, Boulain T, Morawiec E, Cottereau A, Devaquet J, Nseir S, Razazi K, Mira JP, Argaud L, Chakarian J C, Ricard J D, Wittebole X, Chevalier S, Herbland A, Fartoukh M, Constantin JM, Tonnelier J M, Pierrot M, Mathonnet A, Béduneau G, Delétage-Métreau C, Richard J C, Brochard L, Robert R; FLORALI Study Group and the REVA Network. 2015. High-flow oxygen through nasal cannula in acute hypoxemic respiratory failure. *N Engl J Med* 372:2185-96. DOI: 10.1056/NEJMoa1503326.

[2] Li J, Jing G, Scott J B. 2020. Year in Review 2019: High-flow nasal cannula oxygen therapy for adult subjects. *Respir. Care* 65:545–57. DOI:10.4187/respcare.07663.

[3] Mikalsen I B, Davis P, Øymar K. 2016. High flow nasal cannula in children: a literature review. *Scand. J. Trauma Resusc. Emerg. Med.* 24:93. DOI:10.1186/s13049-016-0278-4.

[4] Nishimura M. 2019. High-flow nasal cannula oxygen therapy devices. *Respir. Care* 64:735–42. DOI:10.4187/respcare.06718.

[5] Ritchie J E, Williams A B, Gerard C, Hocke H. 2011. Evaluation of a humidified nasal high-flow oxygen system, using oxygraphy, capnography and measurement of upper airway pressures. *Anaesth. Intensive Care* 39:1103-10. DOI:10.1177/ 0310057x1103900620.

[6] Sun Y H, Dai B, Peng Y, Tan W, Zhao H W. 2019. Factors affecting FiO_2 and PEEP during high-flow nasal cannula oxygen therapy: A bench study. *Clin. Respir. J.* 13:758–764. DOI: 10.1111/crj.13087.

[7] Adams C F, Geoghegan P H, Spence C J, Jermy M C. 2018. Modelling nasal high flow therapy effects on upper airway resistance and resistive work of breathing. *Respir. Physiol. Neurobiol.* 254:23-9. DOI:10.1016/j.resp.2018.03.014.

[8] Möller W, Feng S, Domanski U, Franke KJ, Celik G, Bartenstein, P, Becker S, Meyer G, Schmid O, Eickelberg O, Tatkov S, Nilius G. 2017. Nasal high flow reduces dead space. *J. Appl. Physiol.* 122: 191–7. DOI:10.1152/japplphysiol. 005 84.2016.

[9] Mündel T, Feng S, Tatkov S, Schneider H. 2013. Mechanisms of nasal high flow on ventilation during wakefulness and sleep. *J. Appl. Physiol.* 114:1058–65. DOI:10. 1152/japplphysiol.01308.2012.

[10] Mauri T, Turrini C, Eronia N, Grasselli G, Volta CA, Bellani G, Pesenti A. 2017. Physiologic effects of high-flow nasal cannula in acute hypoxemic respiratory failure. *Am. J. Respir. Crit. Care Med.* 195;1207–15. DOI:10.1164/rccm.201605-0916.

[11] Parke R L, Bloch A, McGuinness S P. 2015. Effect of very-high-flow nasal therapy on airway pressure and end-expiratory lung impedance in healthy volunteers. *Respir. Care*. 60:1397–1403. DOI: 10.4187/respcare.04028.

[12] Groves N, Tobin A. 2007. High flow nasal oxygen generates positive airway pressure in adult volunteers. *Aust. Crit. Care* 20:126—131. DOI:10.1016/j.aucc.20 07.08.001.

[13] Riera J, Pérez P, Cortés J, Roca O, Masclans J R, Rello J. 2013. Effect of high-flow nasal cannula and body position on end-expiratory lung volume: a cohort study using electrical impedance tomography. *Respir. Care* 58:589-96. DOI: 10.4187/respcare. 02086.

[14] Di mussi R, Spadaro S, Stripoli T, Alberto C, Trerotoli P, Pierucci P, Staffieri F, Bruno F, Camporota L, Grasso S. 2018. High-flow nasal cannula oxygen therapy decreases postextubation neuroventilatory drive and work of breathing in patients with chronic obstructive pulmonary disease. *Critical Care* 22:180. DOI:10.1186/ s13054-018-2107-9.

[15] Hochberg CH, Semler MW, Brower RG. 2021. Oxygen Toxicity in Critically Ill Adults. *Am. J. Respir. Crit. Care Med.* 204:632–41. DOI:10.1164/rccm.202102-0417CI.

Chapter 3

Technology and Devices

Diana Amorim*, MD
Pulmonology Clinic, Leiria Hospital Center, Leiria, Portugal

Abstract

High-flow nasal cannula (HFNC) is a non-invasive method that improves patient oxygenation when conventional oxygen therapy is not enough since it provides heated and humidified oxygen able of high flow of up to 60 L/min and 100% of fraction of inspired oxygen (FiO_2). A typical HFNC system consists of a flow generator, active heated humidifier, single-limb heated circuit and nasal cannula. It has great potential for use in a variety of condition, such as hypoxemic respiratory failure, pre-intubation oxygenation, post-extubation, postoperative, palliative care, bronchoscopy, respiratory failure in immunocompromised patients, bronchiectasis and in selected cases of hypercapnic respiratory failure. This chapter summarizes the mechanisms of action and devices of HFNC considering literature.

Keywords: high-flow nasal cannula, respiratory failure, fraction of inspired oxygen, nasal cannula

Overview

When considering hypoxemic respiratory failure, the frontline treatment is supplemental oxygen. Oxygen therapy can be delivered in many ways, ranging

---

* Corresponding Author's Email: dianasofiaamorim@gmail.com.

In: Nasal High Flow and Non-Invasive Ventilatory Support
Editors: A. M. Esquinas, D. A. Lagonidis, P. Silva Santos et al.
ISBN: 979-8-88697-420-1

from conventional oxygen therapy (cannulas and simple oxygen facemask), non-invasive methods and invasive mechanical ventilation (IMV). High-flow nasal cannula (HFNC) is a non-invasive method that improves patient oxygenation when conventional oxygen therapy is not enough since it provides heated and humidified oxygen able of high flow of up to 60 L/min and 100% of fraction of inspired oxygen (FiO_2) [1]. The high flow increases the airway and alveolar pressure, which can create a positive end-expiratory pressure (PEEP) and reduces the dead space by expelling expired gas that has accumulated in the anatomical dead space of the nasopharynx [2].

The mechanisms of action and benefits of HFNC include a range of effects [3, 4]. Clinical gains: patient comfort and tolerability, reduced symptoms of dyspnea and respiratory rate, ease of use.

Physiological impacts: As HFNC is an open system, it does not actively enhance tidal volume, but it improves alveolar ventilation and recruitment by washing out anatomic dead space. It also provides high oxygenation and better control over FiO_2 than standard oxygen systems.

It has great potential for use in a variety of condition, such as hypoxemic respiratory failure, pre-intubation oxygenation, post-extubation, postoperative applications, palliative care, bronchoscopy, respiratory failure in immune-compromised patients, bronchiectasis, and in selected cases of hypercapnic respiratory failure [2, 3].

Technology of High-Flow Nasal Cannula

HFNC devices can be stand-alone units, such as the Optiflow® and the Airvo-2® models or may be integrated within mechanical ventilators. A typical HFNC system consists of a flow generator, active heated humidifier, single-limb heated circuit, and nasal cannula. The flow generator allows a FiO_2 from 21% to 100% and generates up to 60 L/min flow rates. The gas is heated and humidified through a heated humidifier and delivered to the patient via a single limb circuit into though a nasal cannula of large diameter [5]. There is also a water bag that fills the humidifier container, and it must be placed as high as possible above the humidifier to achieve flow of water into the humidifier chamber [5].

Flow Generators

There are three types of flow generators [3, 4].

1) Air-oxygen blenders (the most popular) are supplied by air and oxygen from the divider, regulated by the flow meter, at a low-pressure system. They assure the stable conveyance of FiO_2 and gas stream. Some examples are Fisher & Paykel Healthcare™, Auckland, New Zeeland, Optiflow®.
2) Turbines built in the device (Fisher and & Paykel Healthcare™ Airvo-2®): These are high-flow devices consisting of turbines to entrain room air and generate a high stream in the absence gas supply from the wall or the tank.
3) Entrainment frameworks (Maxtec™, Utah, USA, MaxVenturi®): Deliver high flow and a higher concentration of oxygen.

Humidifiers and Heated Circuits

The cold and dry gas delivered by traditional oxygen systems can lead to airway inflammation, increase resistance, and impair mucociliary function [6]. As in HFNC the flow rates are higher, heated water humidification is necessary to avoid drying of respiratory secretions and to maintain nasal cilia function [5].

In HFNC, humidification is generated by passing blended gas through a bundle of thin tubes with 0.005 pore size [4]. A heated-wire circuit is used to minimize condensation and avoid liquid water from obstructing the HFNC. To regulate the thermal output of the heating wire placed inside the limb, the supplied electric current is servo-controlled [4, 5]. More sophisticated circuits have recently been developed. For example, use of heating wires embedded in the circuit wall keeps the wall temperature high enough to avoid condensation.

We can set humidifier at the desired temperature in our HFNC device, according to the best tolerance and comfort of the patient. For patients with acute hypoxemic respiratory failure there is evidence that lowering the temperature to 31°C can be more comfortable than 37°C [4].

Interface

The interface consists of a special nasal cannula, with a larger diameter and more comfortable than noninvasive positive pressure ventilation (NPPV) [2]. These cannulas can accommodate a high inlet flow of at least 60 L/min. The nasal prongs are held in place on the upper lip with an elastic over-ear and head band. There also are adapters for tracheostomized patients [5]. Do not forget to select appropriate size nasal cannula and circuit tubing for patient size, since prongs should not totally occlude nares.

The Optiflow® system (Fisher & Paykel) is the most well-known. The nasal prongs and tubing between the nasal prong and inspiratory circuit are both large bore, and flow to the prongs is delivered from one side only. It has a concave base designed to alleviate pressure on the septum and permeable membrane allows water vapor to diffuse through the walls of the tubing freely. Anatomical design to improve airflow and sit comfortably in the nares.

Fraction of Inspired Oxygen

We need to use oxygen flow meters (0-70 L/min) to regulate FiO_2 that we want to give to the patient [5]. In some devices it is possible to see directly in the screen the FiO_2 we are offer, while in other ones we must calculate manually, as in the equation bellow:

$$\% FiO2 = \frac{O2\ Flow \times 100 + (Turbine\ Flow - O2\ Flow) \times 21}{Turbine\ Flow}$$

The required oxygen concentration differs among patients. Adjust the fraction of inspired oxygen (FiO_2) after setting the flow rate to accommodate mixed gas leakage during inspiration. Adjust the oxygen saturation to 94–98% for type I respiratory failure and to 88–92% for type II respiratory failure.

With higher inspiratory flow rates there is a limitation of heating and humidifying of inspired oxygen as well as increased entrainment of room air, which leads to dilution of oxygen [1]. This means that if we increase the inspiratory flow rate, we are going to lower FiO_2. As FIO_2 increases, air entrainment also decreases; however, the required rise in oxygen flow to keep the total flow constant also generates more noise and louder noise increases patient discomfort [2, 4, 7]. Also, we should consider that patients with more-severe hypoxemia find higher flows more comfortable, so it is important to consider a balance of all these parameters.

Devices of High-Flow Nasal Cannula

There are a lot of different devices in the market, but few studies have compared differences of each other (by the flow and FiO_2, for example). A study performed in China in 2020 compared four HFNC devices (AIRVO 2, TNI softFlow 50, HUMID-BH, and OH-70C) and a ventilator with an HFNC module (bellavista 1000), concluding that AIRVO 2 and OH-70C showed better FiO_2 accuracy. TNI softFlow 50, bellavista 1000, and HUMID-BH could lower the risk of insufficient flow support due to accidental compression, bending, or blocking of the nasal cannulas [8]. In the future, more studies will be necessary in this area.

References

[1] Ischaki E, Pantazopoulos I, Zakynthinos S. Nasal high flow therapy: A novel treatment rather than a more expensive oxygen device. *Eur. Respir. Rev.* 2017; 26(145). doi:10.1183/16000617.0028-2017.

[2] Simon Oczkowski, Begüm Ergan, Lieuwe Bos, Michelle Chatwin, Miguel Ferrer, Cesare Gregoretti, Leo Heunks, Jean-Pierre Frat, Federico Longhini, Stefano Nava, Paolo Navalesi, Aylin Ozsancak Uğurlu, Lara Pisani, Teresa Renda, Arnaud W Thille, João Carlos Winck, Wolfram Windisch, Thomy Tonia, Jeanette Boyd, Giovanni Sotgiu, Raffaele Scala. ERS clinical practice guidelines: high-flow nasal cannula in acute respiratory failure. *Eur. Respir. J.* 2022;59(4). doi:10.1183/13993003.01574-2021.

[3] Miguel Guia, Nilgun Alpay, António Gerardo, Yasmin Madney, Mohamed Abdelrahim, Haitham Saeed, Hadeer Harb, Gil Gonçalves, Bruno Cabrita, Jaber Alqahtani, Mohamad El-Khatib, Manuel Gómez-Ríos, Atefeh Fakharian, Laura Ciobanu, Habib Md Reazaul Karim, Edoardo Piervincenzi, Martin Scharffenberg, Paschalis Steiropoulos, William LeMaster, Igor Barjaktarevic, Jakob Wittenstein, Montserrat Diaz-Abad, Andreas Perren, Antonello Nicolini, Savino Spadaro, Giancarlo Garuti, Angelo Petroianni, Antonio Esquinas· High-flow nasal oxygen therapy in acute hypoxemic respiratory failure: Concise review on technology and initial methodology. *Turkish Thorac. J.* 2021;22(6):494-500. doi:10.5152/TurkThoracJ.2021.20213.

[4] Nishimura M. High-flow nasal cannula oxygen therapy devices. *Respir. Care.* 2019;64(6):735-742. doi:10.4187/respcare.06718.

[5] Goteraa C, Díaz Lobato S, Pinto T, Winck JC. Clinical evidence on high flow oxygen therapy and active humidification in adults. *Rev. Port Pneumol.* 2013; 19(5):217-227. doi:10.1016/j.rppnen.2013.03.006.

[6] Lodeserto F J, Lettich T M, Rezaie S R. High-flow Nasal Cannula: Mechanisms of Action and Adult and Pediatric Indications. *Cureus.* 2018;10(11). doi:10.7759/ cureus.3639.

[7] Jean-Pierre Frat, Arnaud W Thille, Alain Mercat, Christophe Girault, Stéphanie Ragot, Sébastien Perbet, Gwénael Prat, Thierry Boulain, Elise Morawiec, Alice Cottereau, Jérôme Devaquet, Saad Nseir, Keyvan Razazi, Jean-Paul Mira, Laurent Argaud, Jean-Charles Chakarian, Jean-Damien Ricard, Xavier Wittebole, Stéphanie Chevalier, Alexandre Herbland, Muriel Fartoukh, Jean-Michel Constantin, Jean-Marie Tonnelier, Marc Pierrot, Armelle Mathonnet, Gaëtan Béduneau, Céline Delétage-Métreau, Jean-Christophe M Richard, Laurent Brochard, René Robert, FLORALI Study Group; REVA Network. High-Flow Oxygen through Nasal Cannula in Acute Hypoxemic Respiratory Failure. *N. Engl. J. Med.* 2015; 372(23):2185-2196. doi:10.1056/nejmoa1503326.

[8] Zhou Y, Ni Z, Ni Y, Liang B, Liang Z. Comparison of Actual Performance in the Flow and Fraction of Inspired O2among Different High-Flow Nasal Cannula Devices: A Bench Study. *Can. Respir. J.* 2021;2021. doi:10.1155/2021/6638048.

Chapter 4

Non-Invasive Ventilation: Options and Methodology

Christos Triantafyllou[1,*], RN and Pavlos Myrianthefs[2,3], MD

[1] Center for Clinical Epidemiology and Outcomes Research (CLEO), Non-Profit Civil Partnership, Neo Psichiko, Athens, Greece
[2] National and Kapodistrian University of Athens, School of Health Sciences, Department of Nursing, Papadiamantopoulou, Goudi, Athens, Greece
[3] "Agioi Anargyroi" General Hospital, Nea Kifissia, Greece

Abstract

Non-invasive ventilation (NIV) refers to the provision of ventilation support without the use of an invasive artificial airway (endotracheal tube or tracheostomy tube). The use of NIV has significantly increased over the last two decades, and NIV is now an essential tool in the management of acute and chronic respiratory failure in both the home, emergency, and critical care settings.

Non-invasive positive pressure ventilation (NIPPV) refers to the delivery of mechanical ventilation to the lungs using techniques that do not require an endotracheal tube. Bilevel positive airway pressure (BiPAP) is the most common mode of NIPPV and requires provisions for inspiratory positive airway pressure (IPAP) and expiratory positive airway pressure (EPAP). In the past decade, NPPV has gained wide acceptance and is now used more frequently after the development of portable ventilators, new modes of ventilation, and other equipment. NIV support uses a variety of interfaces, and these interfaces continue to

* Corresponding Author's Email: christrian@nurs.uoa.gr.

In: Nasal High Flow and Non-Invasive Ventilatory Support
Editors: A. M. Esquinas, D. A. Lagonidis, P. Silva Santos et al.
ISBN: 979-8-88697-420-1

evolve with modifications based on patient comfort and efficiency. Many of the interfaces or masks were initially used in patients with obstructive sleep apnea before being adapted for patient use to provide NIV support. Nasal and orofacial masks were the first interfaces, followed by the development and use of full-face masks, mouthpieces, nasal pillows, and helmets. Nasal masks and orofacial masks are still the most used interfaces.

Adequate ventilation and oxygenation, correction of respiratory failure, and appropriate patient tolerance and comfort are the primary goals of non-invasive ventilation, and adjustments are made to achieve these endpoints. Identifying patients who are proper candidates for NIV and those for whom NIV is unlikely to be effective can help avoid inappropriate NIV application or unnecessary delays before invasive ventilation is initiated. Objective criteria for discontinuation are important to limit trials to patients in whom non-invasive ventilation ultimately fails.

Keywords: bilevel positive airway pressure, inspiratory positive airway pressure, expiratory positive airway pressure, masks, interfaces

Introduction

Non-invasive ventilation (NIV) refers to the provision of ventilation support without the use of an invasive artificial airway (endotracheal or tracheostomy tubes). The use of NIV has significantly increased over the last two decades, and NIV is now an essential tool in the management of acute and chronic respiratory failure in both home and critical care settings. NIV is used in place of invasive ventilation and, due to its flexibility, is also a valuable complement to patient management. Its use in acute respiratory failure is widely accepted and widespread [1].

Although, the role of NIV in patients with chronic respiratory failure is less clear and has not yet been defined [2]. In this chapter, NIV is discussed in terms of options and methodology of delivery.

Options and Methodology of Delivery

Non-Invasive Positive-Pressure Ventilation (NIPPV)

NIPPV with a mask has become the primary method of providing NIV support and is the focus of this and subsequent sections. Early bedside physiologic studies of healthy patients and patients with respiratory disorders documented successful ventilatory support (i.e., decreased respiratory rate, increased tidal volume, decreased dyspnea) with a reduction in diaphragmatic electromyography (EMG), transdiaphragmatic pressure, work of breathing and improvement in oxygenation with a reduction of hypercapnia [3].

Ventilation support can be achieved through different interfaces (mouthpiece, nasal, face, or helmet mask), using a variety of ventilation modes (e.g., volume ventilation, pressure support, bilevel positive airway pressure (BiPAP), proportional-assist ventilation (PAV), continuous positive airway pressure (CPAP) with either ventilator suitable for NIV or ventilators capable of supporting through an endotracheal tube or mask. Older models of non-invasive ventilators required oxygen to be supplied to the system, but current models merge oxygen blenders for precise administration of the fraction of inspired oxygen (FIO_2) [4].

Non-Invasive Negative-Pressure Ventilation (NINPV)

NINPV can be administrated using a device that wraps around the thoracic cage starting from the neck, and devices vary from a full-body tank to a cuirass shell. The general principle is the same as the vacuum device, which reduces the pressure surrounding the thorax, creating sub-atmospheric pressure, and thus passively expanding the chest wall with diaphragmatic descent, which leads to an inflation of the lung. Exhalation occurs with passive recoil of the chest wall [5]. This was the dominant technology during the poliomyelitis epidemic, but these devices were cumbersome and difficult to use.

Upper airway obstruction is also a problem. These ventilators have been largely replaced by the more widespread non-invasive positive pressure ventilation (NIPPV). However, some patients continue to be treated with this modality. While most experience has been in patients with chronic respiratory failure, especially neuromuscular respiratory failure, reports have described successful application in patients with acute respiratory failure [5].

As for the two modes, positive-pressure ventilation has replaced negative-pressure ventilation as the predominant NIV mode. Positive-pressure ventilation is more effective than negative-pressure ventilation in unloading the respiratory muscles, at least under experimental conditions.

High-Flow Nasal Oxygen

As a result of prospective, randomized clinical trials, another option has emerged for patients with hypoxemic respiratory failure. Heated, humidified, high-flow nasal cannula oxygen supplementation (HFNC) has been around for more than a decade, but technical improvements and increasing clinical experience have made it a solid alternative for the management of multiple conditions instead of the application of non-non-invasive or invasive mechanical ventilation. This modality was originally developed for neonatal patients, and improvements have allowed being used in adults.

Conventional oxygen therapy is not well tolerated at high flow rates due to problems with unheated, non-dehumidified oxygen. The HFNC oxygen system provides heating and humidification, improving patient tolerance and comfort. The high flow rates have other advantages in that high flow rates minimize room air entrainment, thereby increasing the FiO_2 that can be provided to patients; are able to wash out dead space carbon dioxide, improving the efficiency of oxygen delivery; and the increased flow rate translates into low level positive end-expiratory pressures (PEEP). The amount of PEEP provided is a function of the flow rate but falls somewhere in the range of 0.35-0.69cm water for each 10L/min of increased flow rate [6].

Thus, although HFNC devices technically do not provide the same assisted support or augment inspired tidal volume as the other forms of mechanical ventilation, a small amount of positive pressure provided does help reduce the work of breathing and improve breathing patterns in a manner similar to that achieved with CPAP. This modality requires an intact airway, which means it is not suitable for patients with hypoventilation or an obstructed airway. It is reasonable to consider this modality as a method of providing low-level positive pressures and PEEP. However, it is not assisted ventilation, at its most rudimentary, it is a form of NIV.

HFCN oxygen seems especially suited to the recently extubated, postoperative patient and those with mild-to-moderate acute hypoxemic respiratory failure, as may occur in patients with decompensated heart failure [7].

Methodology NIV Application

Location of Application

1 It can be used in the ICU, especially if there is a possibility of intubation.

2 It can be used in a step-down unit (lower severity of illness), as follows:
- Moderately severe COPD (pH >7.30).
- Do-not-intubate status.
- Intermittent or nocturnal ventilatory support.

3 It can be used in the ward setting (not recommended if intubation is a consideration) [8].

Patient Interfaces

In the simplest terms, NIV differs from invasive ventilation by the interface between the patient and the ventilator. Invasive ventilation support is provided via either an endotracheal tube or a tracheostomy tube. NIV support uses a variety of interfaces, and these interfaces continue to evolve with modifications based on patient comfort and efficiency. Many of the interfaces or masks were initially used in patients with obstructive sleep apnea (OSA) before being adapted for patient use to provide NIV support. Nasal and orofacial masks were the first interfaces, followed by the development and use of full-face masks, mouthpieces, nasal pillows, and helmets. Nasal masks and orofacial masks are still the most used interfaces. Orofacial masks are used almost twice as frequently as nasal masks. Both have advantages and disadvantages in the application of non-invasive ventilation (Table 1) [9].

The fit of the mask or other interface is another key element of successful NIV. The mask or interface may be kept in place (without the straps) by the patient or therapist to familiarize the patient with the mask and ventilator. As a rule, the smallest mask providing proper fit is the most effective. The straps hold the mask in place, taking care to minimize excess pressure on the face or nose. Leakage is a limitation of all the interfaces, but excessive pressure applied with the straps increases the risk of pressure necrosis and skin breakdown (pressure ulcers). The straps should be tight enough to prevent leaks but loose enough that a finger or two can slip between the face and the straps [9].

The nasal and orofacial masks may be first-line and second-line options, especially in patients who may have prior knowledge of these interfaces or in those who may have had difficulty with nasal or orofacial masks. Clinical trials have not demonstrated the superiority of any mask, although nasal masks may be more effective in patients with less severe diseases. In patients with higher severity of illness, the orofacial mask and total face mask appear to have comparable outcomes. The main considerations when choosing a nasal or orofacial mask are outlined below [9]. Advantages of orofacial mask:

- Best suited for less cooperative patients.
- Better in patients with higher severity of illness.
- Better for patients with mouth-breathing or pursed-lips breathing.
- Better in edentulous patients.
- Generally, more effective ventilation.

Cautions and disadvantages of orofacial mask:

- Claustrophobic.
- Hinder speaking and coughing.
- Risk of aspiration with emesis.

Advantages of nasal mask:

- Best suited for more cooperative patients.
- Better in patients with lower severity of illness.
- Not claustrophobic.
- Allows speaking, drinking, coughing, and secretion clearance.
- Less aspiration risk with emesis.
- Generally, better tolerated.

Cautions and disadvantages of nasal mask:

- More leaks are possible (e.g., mouth-breathing or edentulous patients).
- Effectiveness is limited in patients with nasal deformities or blocked nasal passages.

While orofacial and nasal masks are the most used interfaces, other patient-ventilator interfaces through which non-invasive ventilation can be applied include mouthpieces, nasal pillows, total face masks, and even helmet devices that cover the entire head. Experience with helmet devices is limited but increasing, and it has been successful in patients unable to tolerate nasal or orofacial devices [9]. Summary in Table 1.

Table 1. Advantages and disadvantages of orofacial and nasal mask

Orofacial mask	
Advantages	*Disadvantages*
Best suited for less cooperative patients	Claustrophobic
Better in patients with a higher severity of illness	Hinder speaking and coughing
Better for patients with mouth-breathing or pursed-lips breathing	Risk of aspiration with emesis
Better in edentulous patients	
Subsequent adjustments based on arterial blood gas values	
Advantages	*Disadvantages*
Best suited for more cooperative patients	More leaks possible
Better in patients with a lower severity of illness	Effectiveness limited in patients with nasal deformities or blocked nasal passages
Not claustrophobic	
Allows speaking, drinking, coughing, and secretion clearance	
Less aspiration risk with emesis	
Generally better tolerated	

Ventilators

The choice of ventilators available to provide NIV support has continued to expand. Early NIV support was applied using either a bedside large critical care volume ventilator or a dedicated smaller volume or pressure ventilator specifically developed for NIV. While intensive care ventilators have more options, they are also less tolerant of leaks. The specialty ventilators had fewer options and range, but they were more leak tolerant [10].

Many critical care ventilators currently in use also have the option of NIV, either as part of the original device or available as an upgrade option. The ideal device is dependent on a number of factors, including familiarity by the medical and nursing staff and available options. The distinction between the bedside critical care ventilators and specialty non-invasive ventilator continue to shrink as differences in ventilator options, range of support, and leak tolerance are corrected in both devices. The distinction between functions and capabilities has been blurred, and there are devices that can provide both invasive ventilation and NIV with a simple change of ventilator settings. However, most hospitals continue to provide non-invasive support with the specialized smaller ventilators [10].

Modes of Ventilation

The selection of the initial ventilation mode is partly based on past experience, partly on the support capacity of available ventilators, and partly on the condition being treated. Most patients receiving NIV are provided support with pressure ventilation, with CPAP being the most basic level of support. CPAP may be particularly helpful in patients with congestive heart failure or obstructive sleep apnea [10].

BiPAP is probably the most common mode NIPPV and requires provisions for inspiratory positive airway pressure (IPAP) and expiratory positive airway pressure (EPAP). The distinction between IPAP and EPAP reflects the amount of pressure support ventilation delivered to the patient, and EPAP is synonymous with PEEP. Some NIV is provided using PAV, which supports flow and volume during each breath. Clinical trials have failed to demonstrate a significant difference between PAV and pressure-support ventilation with BiPAP. However, BiPAP is the most common and frequently used modality for NIV. PAV remains available on many ventilator models, but its use is much less common than with BiPAP [10].

While volume ventilators can be used to provide NIV support, the modes described previously are preferred because they provide better patient comfort and synchronization and are more tolerant of the leaks that accompany all NIV interfaces [11].

Initial Ventilator Settings and Adjustments

Adequate ventilation and oxygenation, correction of respiratory failure, and appropriate patient tolerance and comfort are the primary goals of non-invasive ventilation, and adjustments are made to achieve these endpoints. These initial settings focus on achieving adequate V_t, typically around 5-7mL/kg. Additional support is given to reduce the respiratory rate to less than

25 breaths/min. Oxygen is adjusted to achieve adequate oxygenation, with a pulse oximetry goal of over 90% [12].

Serial arterial blood gas measurements are necessary to monitor the response to therapy and to guide subsequent ventilator settings. In patients who may benefit from non-invasive chronic non-invasive support, baseline values should be based on prior support levels. The listed levels may not be sufficient and will therefore increase the likelihood of intolerance or failure. If there is uncertainty, it is important to perform a bedside titration with increasing levels based on patient comfort or exhaled V_t. These adjustments can be made within minutes and can be done without obtaining blood gases (Table 2) [12].

Table 2. Initial ventilator settings and adjustments

Initial IPAP/EPAP settings
Start at 10 cmH_2O/5 cmH_2O.
Pressures less than 8cmH_2O/4cm H_2O not advised as this may be inadequate.
Initial adjustments to achieve Vt of 5-7 mL/kg (IPAP and/or EPAP).
Nasal mask
Increase IPAP by 2 cm H_2O if persistent hypercapnia.
Increase IPAP and EPAP by 2 cm H_2O if hypoxemia persists.
Maximal IPAP limited to 20-25 cm H_2O (avoids gastric distension, improves patient comfort)
Maximal EPAP limited to 10-15 cm H_2O.
FiO_2 at 1.0 and adjust to lowest level with an acceptable pulse oximetry value.
Back up respiratory rate 12-16 breaths/min.
Increase IPAP by 2 cm H_2O if hypercapnia persists.

IPAP, inspiratory positive airway pressure; EPAP, and expiratory positive airway pressure.

Initial IPAP/EPAP settings are:

- Start at 10cm H_2O/5cmH_2O.
- Pressures less than 8cm H_2O/4cm H_2O not advised as this may be inadequate.
- Initial adjustments to achieve Vt of 5-7mL/kg (IPAP and/or EPAP).

Subsequent adjustments based on arterial blood gas values are:

- Increase IPAP by 2 cmH_2O if persistent hypercapnia.
- Increase IPAP and EPAP by 2 cmH_2O if persistent hypoxemia.

- Maximal IPAP limited to 20-25 cmH_2O (avoids gastric distension, improves patient comfort).
- Maximal EPAP limited to 10-15 cmH_2O.
- FiO_2 at 1.0 and adjust to lowest level with an acceptable pulse oximetry value.
- Back up respiratory rate 12-16 breaths/min.

Predictors of Success and Failure of NIV

It is important to recognize that certain parameters may predict successful non-invasive ventilation or failure of non-invasive ventilation, so that patients are not treated as continuously when optimal treatment requires invasive mechanical ventilation.

This includes changes during a trial of NIV. The changes, in turn, reflect the patient's ability to cooperate with non-invasive ventilation, patient-ventilatory synchronization, and the effectiveness of NIV. Trials of NIV typically last 12 hours and are helpful in determining if a patient can be treated with non-invasive ventilation.

Extended trials without significant improvement are not recommended as these only delay intubation and mechanical ventilation (unless patients are do-not-intubate status) [13].

Predictors of success with a response to a trial of NIV (1-2h) are:

- Decrease in $PaCO_2$ greater than 8mmHg.
- Improvement in pH greater than 0.06.
- Correction of respiratory acidosis.

Predictors of failure are:

- The severity of illness - Acidosis ($pH < 7.25$), hypercapnia (>80 and $pH < 7.25$), Acute Physiology and Chronic Health Evaluation II (APACHE II) score higher than 20.
- Level of consciousness - Neurologic score (>4 = stuporous, arousal only after vigorous stimulation; inconsistently follows commands), encephalopathy score (>3 = major confusion, daytime sleepiness, or agitation), Glasgow Coma Scale (GCS) score lower than 8 (coma).

- Failure of improvement with 12-24 hours of non-invasive ventilation.

Late admission predictors of failure (>48 h after initiation of non-invasive ventilation) are:

- Lower functional status (Activity score < 2 -> dyspnea light activity).
- Initial acidosis (pH $\leq$7.22).
- Hospital complications (pneumonia, shock, coma).

Certain patients may benefit from a therapeutic trial, however, it is important to limit trials to avoid delays in definitive therapy. Trials may be as short as a few minutes in patients with immediate failure and probably should not exceed 2 hours if the patient does not improve [13].

Objective criteria for discontinuation are important to limit trials to patients in whom non-invasive ventilation ultimately fails. This refers specifically to intubation criteria, which are subjective but have been defined in the international literature in clinical studies. All these criteria are subject to some degree of interpretation in the context of the patient's clinical condition. Importantly, consider the following as a guide to assist with the decision to intubate a patient. Most patients who meet these criteria are candidates for intubation, but a few can be managed with continuous NIV [13].

Conclusion

The use of NIV has significantly increased over the last two decades, and NIV is now an essential tool in the management of acute and chronic respiratory failure in both the home and critical care settings. Non-invasive positive-pressure ventilation (NIPPV) with a mask has become the primary method of providing NIV support.

Identifying patients who are proper candidates for NIV and those for whom NIV is unlikely to be effective can help avoid inappropriate NIV application or unnecessary delays before the initiation of invasive ventilation. Choosing the proper interface and ventilation settings and ensuring close monitoring in the appropriate hospital environment is critical to the success of NIV. Patients at high risk of NIV failure should only be managed by experienced personnel, using an extremely cautious approach to prevent harm.

References

[1] Ozsancak A, Sidhom SS, Liesching TN, Howard W and Hill NS. 2011. "Evaluation of the Total Face Mask for Noninvasive Ventilation to Treat Acute Respiratory Failure."*Chest,* 139 (5): 1034-41. https://doi.org/10.1378/chest.10-1905.

[2] Singh G and Michelle Cao. 2020. "Noninvasive Ventilator Devices and Modes." *Sleep Medicine Clinics,* 15 (4): 545-55. https://doi.org/10.1016/j.jsmc.2020.08.005.

[3] Khan MU. 2011. "Noninvasive Positive Pressure Ventilation in Hospital Setting." *JPMA. The Journal of the Pakistan Medical Association,* 61 (6): 592-97.

[4] Fakharian A and Hill NS. 2013. "NIPPV: Where Are We Now?" *Tanaffos,* 12 (3): 6-8.

[5] Corrado A and Gorini M. 2002. "Long-Term Negative Pressure Ventilation." *Respiratory Care Clinics of North America,* 8 (4): 545-57, v–vi. https://doi.org/10.1016/s1078-5337(02)00026-6.

[6] Parke, Rachael L., and Shay P. McGuinness. 2013. "Pressures Delivered by Nasal High Flow Oxygen during All Phases of the Respiratory Cycle." *Respiratory Care* 58 (10): 1621-24. https://doi.org/10.4187/respcare.02358.

[7] Nishimura M. 2016. "High-Flow Nasal Cannula Oxygen Therapy in Adults: Physiological Benefits, Indication, Clinical Benefits, and Adverse Effects." *Respiratory Care,* 61 (4): 529-41. https://doi.org/10.4187/respcare.04577.

[8] Bello G, De Pascale G and Antonelli M. 2016. "Noninvasive Ventilation." *Clinics in Chest Medicine,* 37 (4): 711-21. https://doi.org/10.1016/j.ccm.2016.07.011.

[9] Mas A and Masip J. 2014. "Noninvasive Ventilation in Acute Respiratory Failure." *International Journal of Chronic Obstructive Pulmonary Disease,* 9: 837-52. https://doi.org/10.2147/COPD.S42664.

[10] Scott JB. 2019. "Ventilators for Noninvasive Ventilation in Adult Acute Care." *Respiratory Care,* 64 (6): 712-22. https://doi.org/10.4187/respcare.06652.

[11] Prasad KT, Gandra RR, Dhooria S, Muthu V, Aggarwal AN, Agarwal R and Sehga IS. 2021. "Comparing Noninvasive Ventilation Delivered Using Neurally-Adjusted Ventilatory Assist or Pressure Support in Acute Respiratory Failure." *Respiratory Care,* 66 (2): 213-20. https://doi.org/10.4187/respcare.07952.

[12] Bello G, Ionescu Maddalena A, Giammatteo V and Antonelli M. 2018. "Noninvasive Options." *Critical Care Clinics,* 34 (3): 395-412. https://doi.org/10.1016/j.ccc.2018.03.007.

[13] Umesh G and Sundararajan L. 2018. "Early Predictors of Success of Non-Invasive Ventilation in Acute Hypercapnic Respiratory Failure." *European Respiratory Journal,* 52 (suppl 62). https://doi.org/10.1183/13993003.congress-2018.PA2352.

Chapter 5

Combined Options of Prone Positioning in Awake Hypoxemic Patients

Giuseppe Fiorentino[1*], MD
Maurizia Lanza[1], MD
Anna Annunziata[1], MD
and Antonio M. Esquinas[2], MD, PhD, FCCP
[1] Unit of Respiratory Physiopathology, Monaldi Hospital, Naples, Italy
[2] Intensive Care Unit, Hospital Morales Meseguer, Murcia, Spain

Abstract

Prone positioning has been utilized for over 40 years to enhance oxygenation in patients needing invasive mechanical ventilation for acute respiratory distress syndrome (ARDS). The first demonstration of an advantageous effect on patient oxygenation was shown in 1974. These results were later documented in several meta-analyses.

Due to the positive physiological effects of prone positioning on transpulmonary pressure, lung compression and ventilatory perfusion ratio, it has also been applied to non-intubated patients with acute respiratory failure (ARF) to improve oxygenation and delay or even avoid the need for invasive ventilation.

During the epidemic of conscious and non-intubated COVID-19 patients, prone positioning was used in emergency wards, medical wards, and sub-intensive care units to relieve pressure in ICUs. Several studies have reported improved oxygenation and respiratory rate during prone positioning. However, the impacts on clinical outcomes, specifically

* Corresponding Author's Email: giuseppefiorentino1@gmail.com.

In: Nasal High Flow and Non-Invasive Ventilatory Support
Editors: A. M. Esquinas, D. A. Lagonidis, P. Silva Santos et al.
ISBN: 979-8-88697-420-1

intubation rates and survival, remain undefined and require further observation and study.

Keywords: ARDS, prone positioning, non-invasive ventilation, high-flow nasal cannula, COVID-19

Introduction

Prone positioning (PP) was first proposed in the 1970s to improve gas exchange in acute respiratory distress syndrome (ARDS) and is currently a non-drug treatment used frequently and whenever possible during invasive mechanical ventilation. Subsequent studies have suggested that prone positioning improves oxygenation in most ARDS patients (70% -80%), increasing the mean PaO_2 / FiO_2 ratio by ± 35 mmHg [1]. Early researchers noted the reduced lung compliance and increased atelectasis that characterized this disease and recommended applying positive end-expiratory pressure (PEEP) to enhance oxygenation.

To additionally reduce atelectasis in injured lungs, Bryan suggested prone positioning, theorizing that prone positioning would decrease pleural pressure gradients and restore ventilation to the dorsal lung parts [2]. The first proof of decreased mortality was reported from the PROSEVA study, in which early and prolonged (at least 16 h) prone positioning sessions were used without improving the frequency of complications and shown to decrease mortality in the control of intubated patients with moderate to severe acute respiratory distress syndrome [3]. Prone positioning was thus designated as a rescue procedure for severe hypoxemia, and earlier research concentrated on specifying the mechanism for better gas exchange. To date, we know that prone positioning decreases mortality in the management of intubated patients with moderate to severe acute respiratory distress syndrome and allows for improved oxygenation by improving the mismatch of the ventilation/perfusion ratio. In managing moderate to severe ARDS, prone positioning is therefore strongly recommended [4].

Combining PP with various non-invasive respiratory support (Non-invasive ventilation - NIV, High-flow nasal cannula - HFNC) in ARDS may result in more acceptable physiological results on ventilation-perfusion mismatch, better drainage for infection-induced ARDS purulent lung and improved homogeneity in ARDS mechanics while receiving positive pressure support. Established on these potential beneficial mechanisms, different studies have been performed to test the hypothesis that early use of PP in combination with NIV or HFNC may avoid the need for intubation in patients with moderate to severe ARDS. Assessments of PP combined with HFNC, or NIV were also performed to improve PaO_2 / FiO_2 versus HFNC or NIV support alone and the safety of PP therapy in awake and non-intubated ARDS patients.

The recent COVID-19 pandemic has led to a sharp increase in hospitalizations for acute respiratory failure [5]. Awake prone positioning has been utilized with the goal of containing ICU admission and mechanical ventilation [6]. In non-COVID-19 acute respiratory failure, studies are restricted to a few small, non-randomized studies and have involved patients with various diseases although the outcomes are interesting with regards to improved oxygenation, especially when combined with non-invasive ventilation or the high-flow nasal cannula. Tolerance of prone positioning with the patient awake and not sedated for a long time is a problem. Larger randomized controlled trials are underway to supply consequences regarding clinical benefit and to define optimized prone positioning regimens. Data on spontaneously breathing patients were restricted to retrospective studies or small prospective cohorts [7], until the recent coronavirus disease 2019 (COVID-19) pandemic outbreak distinguished by increased ARDS and intensive care unit overload (ICU).

Physiopathological Effects of Prone Positioning

Effects on Oxygenation

From the beginning, prone positioning was mainly intended and used as a rescue therapy to relieve life-threatening hypoxemia. In 1988, LANGER et al. reported the results of prone positioning on oxygenation in 13 patients with ARDS secondary to direct lung injury predominantly resulting from pneumonia or aspiration phenomena who received a higher PEEP and a lower FIO2 [8]. In this study, the authors conducted lung computed tomography (CT) scans in two patients in both supine and prone positions. It was therefore reported that, during the supine position, the gas/tissue ratio evaluated on CT scan progressively decreased along the ventral-dorsal gradient in the supine position, revealing a progressive loss of aeration. While with the prone position, the gas/tissue ratio increased towards the dorsal regions, expressing more excellent aeration in these regions. On the other hand, it declined in the ventral regions, which depended on the gravitational force. It is supposed that the modification of oxygenation in the prone position is due to a decrease of the intrapulmonary shunt and derives from the concomitant effect of the growth of aeration in the dorsal lung regions where pulmonary perfusion prevails and of the loss of aeration in the ventral regions. Thus, the decrease in intrapulmonary shunt is due to improved ventilation in well-perfused lung areas [9].

Decreased Lung Compression

The consequences of prone and supine positioning on lung density were reached by Gattinoni et al. [10] by computed tomography, in patients with ARDS. In the supine position, the dorsal part of the lung is condensed by its own weight, the weight of the mediastinum, the abdominal compartment, and the weight of the diaphragm. Prone positioning redistributed lung densities from the dorsal to the ventral regions. This result led to the "sponge lung model," in which ARDS was distinguished by a heavy edematous lung that can be likened to a wet sponge.

By positioning the patient in the prone position, the compression of the lung due to its own weight is decreased through a gravitational redistribution of fluids. In addition, the weight of the mediastinum is supported by the breastbone, the most rigid part of the chest. At the same time, the diaphragm is shifted caudally, reducing the compression of the posterior-caudal lung parenchyma. Finally, in a triangular shaped lung, more parenchyma is included in the dorsal than in the ventral half resulting in a more aerated lung in the prone position [11].

Homogenization of Transpulmonary Pressure

Transpulmonary pressure (PL) is the pressure that relaxes the lung. PL is defined as the difference between airway / alveolar pressure and pleural pressure estimated by esophageal pressure: PL = airway/alveolar pressure − pleural pressure, and during spontaneous breathing, the inspiratory effort exerted by the respiratory muscles further decreases the pleural pressure, resulting in lung ventilation (Figure 1).

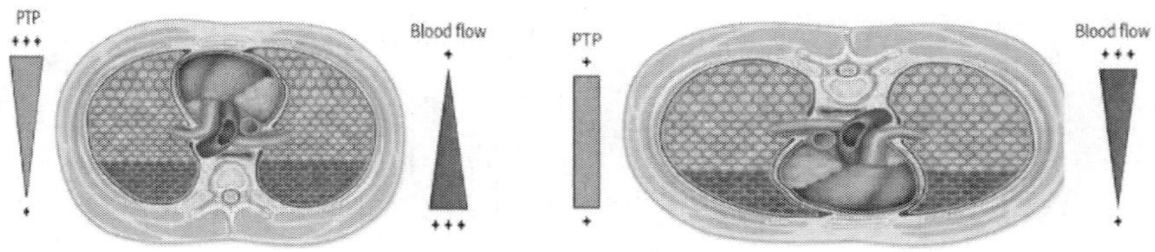

Figure 1. Typical heterogeneous distribution of opacification within the lungs with graphic transpulmonary pressure and blood modifications.

In mechanical ventilation, changes in PL (and changes in lung compliance) are used to define changes in lung volume. For example, for the same level of lung compliance, the higher the PL, the higher the lung volume. The dorsal pleural pressure is greater than the ventral pleural pressure with the patient in the supine position. Consequently, the ventral PL exceeds the dorsal PL. The higher PL in the ventral part of the lung leads to hyperinflation, while the lower PL in the dorsal part of the lung leads to atelectasis [12]. Prone positioning reduces the difference between dorsal and ventral PL, decreasing ventral alveolar hyperinflation and dorsal alveolar collapse.

These mechanisms are increased in ARDS patients, where the dorsal part of the lung is heavier (due to inflammation, edema in the prone areas and weight of the overlying lung), and the tidal volume is preferably distributed to the ventral part, not dependent on the lungs [13].

Ventilation/Perfusion Ratio Improvement

From the work of WEST et al. in 1964 [14] we learned that, in healthy volunteers, pulmonary perfusion is more significant in the lung bases in the upright position and in the dorsal areas of the lung in the supine position. Blood flow is disconnected from the gravitational gradient. In the prone position, the dorsal side continues to receive the most blood flow as the alveoli reopen, while the ventral side continues to receive the least amount of blood flow as the alveoli collapse. Consequently, there is a decrease in the relative intrapulmonary shunt and an improvement in the ventilation/perfusion ratio. In patients with ARDS, the impairment of gas exchange is mainly related to an altered ventilation/perfusion ratio, the management of hypoxemia is geared towards its modification.

Reduction of Ventilator-Induced Lung Injury

In mechanically ventilated patients with ARDS, prone positioning may also control ventilator-induced lung injury (VILI) [15]. VILI includes several pulmonary mechanical changes that can worsen hypoxemia and increase mortality, especially in patients with ARDS. Assuming a protective mechanical ventilation strategy can prevent VILI and enhance survival. This strategy includes an increase in positive end-expiratory pressure (PEEP) to prevent alveolar recruitment and promote over distension of previously well-ventilated alveoli. The acquisition of prone positioning to high PEEP can reduce regional overdistension and small airway opening/closing events, thereby preventing VILI.

Pulmonary overdistension is the first part of VILI, and thus, preventing pulmonary overdistension is the primary concern of intensivists when setting up mechanical ventilation. The second part of VILI is called atelectrauma, which results from repeatedly opening and closing the small airways. Prone positioning causes it to be more homogeneously distributed in the anterior-posterior direction in all lungs: lung density, pulmonary ventilation, intrapulmonary shunt and transpulmonary pressure. By favoring this homogenization, the prone positioning composes the lung to receive the effort imposed by mechanical ventilation. It therefore makes the distribution of the resulting stress more homogeneous through the lung [16].

Stress/strain homogenization is associated with lower VILI risk. Cornejo et al. [17] evaluated supine lung recruitability. The prone position promoted lung recruitment and reduced overdistension in patients in both low and high recruitment categories with low or high PEEP in the prone position. However, tidal recruitment and abandonment, i.e., the cyclic start and closing of small airways (atelectrauma), and tidal hyperinflation were greatly reduced in the prone position only in the subgroup of ARDS patients who had a high recruitability in the supine position and who received higher PEEP levels in the prone position. VILI is underpinned by biochemical and biological events involved in the regulation of lung inflammation a process called biotrauma.

Papazia et al. [18] found that prone position was associated with lower lung concentration of interleukin (IL) -8, IL-6 and IL-1b likened to supine position in ventilated ARDS patients with 6 mL-kg-1 body weight indicated TV and higher PEEP. In rodents undergoing harmful mechanical ventilation (VT 18 mL-kg-1 and PEEP 0 cmH2O), prone ventilation has been established to maintain mitogen-activated protein kinase (MAPK) -phosphatase 1 expression a key regulator in VILI. At the same time, the supine position was associated with significant downregulation. Mice deficient in MAPK-phosphatase 1 were more exposed to VILI. Like intubated ARDS patients, spontaneously breathing patients with hypoxemic ARF can generate advanced respiratory urges and forced inhalation effort, leading to VILI-like lung damage. This concept is called P-SILI and worsens respiratory mechanics and hematosis, directing to an expansion in respiratory drive and an increase in P-SILI, like a vicious cycle. Decreasing inspiratory effort by enhancing gas exchange in the prone position could be an option to reduce P-SILI during ARF [19].

Prone Positioning in Conscious, Non-Intubated, Non-COVID-19 Patients

Evidence of prone positioning benefits in non-intubated patients is limited to a few case reports and small observational studies (Table 1).

Effects on Oxygenation

The first use of prone positioning in spontaneously breathing patients was represented in two studies in 1999 with pediatric patients, in which oxygenation was improved during prone positioning [20]. Two other studies tested awakening prone positioning in patients with severe hypoxemia following lung transplantation, in addendum to non-invasive ventilation (NIV) or high-frequency percussive ventilation. Progress in oxygenation and respiratory mechanics have been reported after multiple sessions [21].

Prone Positioning in Addition to Respiratory Devices

The main goal of NIV and HFNC in ARDS therapy is to achieve sufficient oxygenation to evade endotracheal intubation. However, NIV and HFNC are "partially supportive" therapies only. They do not adequately address the underlying pathology of ARDS, such as the ventilation-perfusion correspondence caused by atelectasis or consolidation independent areas when reinforced with HFNC.

Table 1. Prone positioning in non-intubated, non-COVID-19 patients

First author [ref.]	Patients (n)	Diseases	Respiratory device	PP regimen	Main results	Adverse event	Comments
Chaisupamongkollarp (20)	17	Pneumonia	Oxygen		Improve SpO_2 Improve compliance		Paediatric
Feltracco (21)	2	Post-reimplantation syndrome	NIV	6–8 h per day, 8–10 days	Decrease FIO_2 NIV removal	0	
Feltracco (21)	3	Lung transplant respiratory complications	HFPV	1–3 h, 3–6 times per day	Improve secretions clearance Improve respiratory mechanic Attenuate graft infiltrates Improve gas exchange	0	
Scaravilli (22)	15	Hypoxaemic acute respiratory failure (pneumonia, fascitis, sepsis)	HFNC, CPAP and NIV	3 h per day, 2 days	Improve PaO_2	Intolerance (n=2)	Retrospective PaO_2 return to baseline after resupination
Ding (23)	20	Infectious, moderate-to-severe ARDS (pneumonia, influenza)	NIV and HFNC	30 min twice per day, ≥3 days	Avoid intubation Improve PaO_2 /FIO_2	Intolerance (n=2)	Intubation in 78% of severe ARDS patients

PP: prone positioning; SpO_2: oxygen saturation measured by pulse oximetry; HFNC: high-flow nasal cannula; PaO_2: arterial oxygen tension; CHF: congestive heart failure; ARDS: acute respiratory distress syndrome; NIV: noninvasive ventilation; FIO_2: inspiratory oxygen fraction; HFPV: high-frequency percussive ventilation; CPAP: continuous positive airway pressure

High-level PS combined with deep inspiratory efforts could generate high tidal volumes and excessive transpulmonary pressures, increasing pulmonary stress and contributing to VILI, possibly a risk of NIV insufficiency. A first 5-year retrospective observational study included 15 patients with ARF organized with a high-flow nasal cannula (HFNC) or NIV, who completed multiple prone positioning sessions. The PaO_2 improved significantly during pronation [22].

From the work of Ding et al., the early PP strategy with HFNC or NIV in patients with ARDS caused by an infectious disease proved to be safe and effective in those mild to moderate forms, avoiding intubation in these specific patients. In a second prospective observational study, they recruited 20 patients who similarly received prone positioning in addition to HFNC and NIV for moderate to severe, infectious ARDS [23]. It is a prospective observational study planned to test the hypothesis that early use of PP combined with NIV or HFNC can avoid the need for intubation in patients with moderate to severe ARDS. The effects of PP mixed with HFNC or NIV to improve PaO_2 / FiO_2 versus HFNC or NIV support alone and the safety of PP therapy in awake and non-intubated ARDS patients were also evaluated. The leading cause of ARDS was viral pneumonia, due to the flu (9 cases, 45%) and other viruses (2 cases, 10%). Ten patients fulfilled the criteria for moderate ARDS and ten cases were severe. The primary result for the effectiveness of PP combined with HFNC / NIV was the avoidance rate for intubation. Patients who avoided intubation were classified as successful while those requiring intubation were classified as failure.

The main force of this study is that, for the first time, the early use of PP in combination with HFNC / NIV was considered in awake non-intubated patients with moderate to severe ARDS. This study revealed that early PP combined with HFNC / NIV can avoid the need for intubation in up to half of patients with moderate to severe ARDS; 11 patients avoided intubation, including 8 (73%) moderate ARDS patients and 3 (27%) severe ARDS patients. Nine patients were intubated including 2 (22%) moderate ARDS patients and 7 (78%) severe ARDS patients. Although no difference was statistically significant due to the small sample size of our study, moderate ARDS had a higher percentage in the success group than in the failure group (73% vs 27%, $P = 0.174$. Late acquisition of PP to NIV in severe ARDS carries a high risk of delayed intubation and treatment failure.

Conversely, early application of PP in patients with moderate ARDS and an initial SpO_2 > 95% on NIV may benefit and avoid the need for invasive ventilation. Prone positioning can reduce the need for intubation and even mortality by improving oxygenation of the ARDS. The mean duration of a PP cycle was 2 hours. ARDS was mainly caused by infectious pneumonia and drainage of airway secretions may be important for treatment. Prone positioning in awake patients promotes better airway drainage and, especially if combined with HFNC, may be one of the reasons for avoiding intubation. There are several limitations in this study but firstly, the small sample size that was subject to bias, producing spurious results on statistical analysis It is also unclear whether these advantages persist after resupination and lead to better clinical outcomes.

Prone Positioning in Conscious, Non-Intubated COVID-19 Patients

The COVID-19 pandemic has shown a dramatic growth in the number of patients requiring respiratory support for ARDS, resulting in critical care overload. A large number of COVID-19 patients developed severe bilateral viral pneumonia. Many COVID-19 patients evolve into acute respiratory distress syndrome (ARDS), characterized by profound hypoxemia and an associated high mortality rate.

Nasal high flow oxygen therapy (HFNO) effectively reduces the need for endotracheal intubation in patients with acute hypoxemic respiratory failure (ARF). However, the lack of proven benefits in COVID-19 patients, coupled with concerns of an increased risk of aerosolization, led to advising early intubation and invasive mechanical ventilation (MV) at the start of the pandemic.

Due to the high rate of COVID-19, infection has resulted in a rapid depletion of critical care help around the world. Consequently, physicians had to use innovative strategies to restrict the need for mechanical ventilation, including awake prone positioning. The first benefit of prone positioning in the management of non-intubated COVID patients was shortly described at the start of the pandemic in China, where prone positioning was part of a bundled intervention, including NIV, HFNC, and restrictive fluid resuscitation (Table 2). The authors defined a reduced need for invasive mechanical ventilation, with a lower intubation rate. Regardless, VM is associated with substantial risks including ventilator-associated pneumonia, ICU-acquired weakness, delirium, and cognitive impairment.

Table 2. Prone positioning in non-intubated, COVID-19 patients

First author [ref.]	Design	Patients (n)	Respiratory device	PP regimen	Main results	Adverse event	Comments
Sun (6)	Retrospective analysis	631	HFNC and NIV	Unknown	Combined strategy including PP might decrease mortality		Bundled intervention PP regimen undisclosed
Elharrar (26)	Prospective feasibility study	24	COT and HFNC	≥3 h, one session	Increased PaO2 during PP	Back pain (42%)	3 patients maintained improvement after resupination
Despres (27)	Prospective feasibility study	6	COT and HFNC	1 to 16 h	Improve PaO2/FIO2		In ICU 3 (50%) patients required intubation
Ng (28)	Prospective case series	10	COT	1 h, 5 times per day	Shortening of oxygen weaning	Musculoskelatal discomfort and nausea/vomiting	8 patients received COVID-19 specific therapies
Reddy (29)	Meta-analysis	449	COT, HFNC and NIV	Heterogeneous	Improve oxygenation	Decrease RR	Included 15 studies
Sartini (30	Prospective case series	15	CPAP	Based on severity and adherence	Improve SpO2 and PaO2/FIO2	Decrease RR	80% of patients maintain oxygenation improvement after resupination
Caputo (32)	Observational cohort study	50	COT	5 min.	Improve SpO2		In ED 13 (25%) patients required intubation within 24 h
Thompson (33)	Prospective feasibility study	25	COT	1 h	Improve SpO2		In IMCU 12 (48%) patients required intubation Patients with an SpO2 ≥95% after 1 h of PP was associated with a lower rate of intubation
Hallifax (34)	Retrospective cohort study	30	HFNC and NIV	2 h twice per day, 2 consecutive days			Reduced mortality In ICU only 11 patients "fully" prone
Padrão (35)	Retrospective cohort study	57	COT	≥4 h	Do not reduce intubation rate	Accidental removal of i.v. lines	Only COT was used while other respiratory devices might improve outcomes
Ferrando (36)	Prospective cohort study	55	HFNC	16 h per day	Do not reduce intubation rate		In ICU did not establish whether was used as a routine or life-saving therapy Non-prone group also included regimen <16 h per day
Ferrando (36)	Prospective cohort study	55	HFNC	16 h per day	Do not reduce intubation rate		In ICU did not establish whether was used as a routine or life saving therapy Non-prone group also included regimen <16 h per dey

PP: prone positioning; HFNC: high-flow nasal cannula; NIV: noninvasive ventilation; COT: conventional oxygen therapy; PaO2: arterial oxygen tension; FIO2: inspiratory oxygen fraction; ICU: intensive care unit; SpO2: oxygen saturation measured by pulse oximetry; RR: respiratory rate; CPAP: continuous positive airway pressure; ED: emergency department; IMCU: Intermediate care unit.

The awards, that the potential benefits of HFNC for preventing intubation and protecting critical resources in the ICU, could outweigh its risks soon led to expert guidelines and suggestions supporting its use during the pandemic [24]. Several studies have indicated that the variety of awake PP and HFNO or non-invasive ventilation (NIV) is possible in patients with severe COVID-19 pneumonia, resulting in improved oxygenation or reduced respiratory rate and / or dyspnea [25] (Table 2).

Effects on Oxygenation

Elharrar et al. showed a single-center prospective study of prone positions in patients with hypoxemic ARF needing oxygen supplementation with HFNC or COT [26]. Of the 24 patients included, 15 (63%) accepted an initial prone positioning session for at least 3 hours. Between tolerant patients, PaO_2 increased from 73.6 mmHg earlier to 94.9 mmHg during prone positioning. Only three patients maintained improved oxygenation 6-12 hours after resupination [27, 28]. In hospitalized COVID-19 patients, other similar studies reported improved oxygenation during prone positioning, with a heterogeneous prone positioning regimen. A total of 15 studies, representing 449 patients, were included in a systematic review and meta-analysis, considering the change in oxygenation (i.e., PaO_2 / FIO_2 ratio, PaO_2 and measurement of oxygen saturation by pulse oximetry (SpO_2) after prone positioning [29]. Despite the heterogeneity in the prone positioning regimens and associated respiratory devices, significant improvement in oxygenation was reported at the end of the prone positioning session.

Prone Positioning in Addition to Respiratory Devices

It has been indicated that the prone awake position in spontaneously breathing non-intubated patients with acute respiratory failure enhances oxygenation and was possible in up to 95% of patients. Several small observational studies in COVID-19 patients have documented similar results in patients with spontaneous awake breathing, leading to a recent consensus statement for the management of COVID-19 pneumonia that agreed on the role of the prone position as an adjunct therapy for the treatment of patients who require additional oxygenation to maintain oxygen saturation above 90%.

In complement to the prone position, non-invasive respiratory supports, such as HFNC, CPAP helmet and pressure support, were involved to both improve gas exchange and reduce inspiratory effort. In Italian studies, prone positioning was also utilized in addition to NIV / continuous positive airway pressure (CPAP). In the first, 15 patients who were hypoxemic despite a 10 cmH_2O CPAP were placed prone [30]. All patients enhanced SpO_2, PaO_2 / FIO_2 ratio and respiratory rate. Most of them supported the improvement in oxygenation after prone placement. Besides the CPAP helmet, prone positioning was used for a minimum duration of 3 hours. The PaO_2 / FIO_2 ratio significantly improved, and the improvement was maintained in half of the patients after resupination.

The mixture of prone position and non-invasive respiratory support has been reported to improve oxygenation in most studies. The larger series published by Coppo et al., Which enrolled 56 patients [25] most of them with helmet CPAP, showed that oxygenation enhanced on average by more than 50%. In the present study, oxygenation improved similarly, regardless of their degree of baseline hypoxemia, instantly after 3 h of pronation. This indicates that pronation can be used as an effective strategy that can improve gas exchange as lifesaving or long-term treatment. The study conducted by Chiummello D. et al., evaluated the effect of prone position in wakefulness in COVID19-associated ARDS (CARDS) patients treated with helmet CPAP, showed that the prone position was associated with: (1) a reduction work of breathing, (2) an improvement in oxygenation in 85% of patients, and (3) a reduced sensation of dyspnea in all patients.

Several beneficial mechanisms associated with the prone position previously described in both acute respiratory failure and ARDS could also be found in patients with CARDS. Compatible with previous descriptions, in the initial phase of the disease, lung weight and lung gas volume of patients with CARDS were approximately half and twice that observed in classical ARDS, respectively. The prone position allocated concomitantly with the CPAP helmet, thus, has unique advantages regarding the modification of gas exchange and a reduction in respiratory work, while its impact on endotracheal intubation and invasive mechanical ventilation requirements remains unclear. Possible limits of this study are:

(1) The long-term consequences of the prone position, and the persistence of effects after returning to the supine position are undefined.

(2) The transdiaphragmatic pressure was not calculated, thus the possible effect of expiratory muscle activity on pressure cannot be assessed.
(3) Due to the study design, the effects of prone position on clinically relevant results could not be evaluated.
(4) Prone position was not randomized.

In summary, the prone - awake position in addition to helmet CPAP can be offered to CARDS patients to improve oxygenation and decrease work of breathing (WOB). Nevertheless, rigorous clinical evaluation should succeed in preventing delays in endotracheal intubation and provision of invasive mechanical ventilation [31].

Tolerance of Prone Positioning as a Prognostic Factor

Few studies have reported a possible role of the prone position as a prognostic factor for COVID-19 patients. The first retrospective study was conducted in an emergency room in New York City (NY, USA) and interested 50 patients with hypoxia at triage. The authors documented a significant increase in SpO_2 during prone positioning [32]. Defeat to improve oxygenation during initial proning occurred to be associated with an improved risk of intubation. In the second study, 25 hypoxemic patients in an intermediate care unit had a considerable increase in SpO_2 during prone positioning. A lower rate of intubation was observed in patients with 95% SpO_2 after 1 hour of proning [33]. In addition, recently a retrospective study included 48 patients requiring CPAP and/or HFNC. Only 11 patients could tolerate prone positioning for at least 2 hours twice a day for two successive days (complete proning), but the attainment of full proning was associated with reduced mortality [34].

Effects on Clinical Outcomes

Several studies have particularly investigated whether the use of prone positioning is associated with better clinical outcomes and particularly reduced intubation rate [35]. A single-center retrospective study compared awake prone positioning with routine care in 57 hypoxemic patients who had increased work of breathing (i.e., tachypnea $\geqslant$24 breaths · min − 1). Exposure to prone-awake positioning was not associated with a reduction in intubation rate. Thus [36], (in a prospective multicenter study, prone positioning was employed as an adjunct to HFNC in 55 patients compared with 144 patients. The rate of intubation was not lower in the prone group, but prone positioning was only considered when applied for ⩾16.

In a bi-center exposed / unexposed retrospective matched cohort study, PRUD'HOMME et al. included 96 COVID-19 patients with acute hypoxemic respiratory failure requiring supplemental oxygen. Prone positioning for at least 3 hours a day for three successive days can be associated with clinical benefit by keeping the oxygen delivery method updated. Several conclusions can be drawn with caution from these early studies in COVID-19: prone positioning improves oxygenation during prone position. Scientific proof on the predictive value of initial waking prone arrangement and clinical outcomes is limited and requires future studies.

Clinical Problems and Limitations

Before the first prone positioning session, the patient must explain the method. Make sure respiratory devices and intravenous lines are safe. For the first session, careful initial monitoring (SpO_2 and respiratory rate) should be done. A call bell should be available. Frequent repositioning could increase tolerance. The cushions can be used to improve comfort. A nurse or physical therapist can help with the placement. The application of prone positioning in awake and spontaneously breathing patients has not been extensively investigated. Some limitations can be identified.

Prone positioning in conscious patients could be a complementary tool for improving oxygenation beyond respiratory devices such as COT, HFNC, CPAP or NIV. Numerous studies have shown that prone placement improves oxygenation, at least during prone placement. Nevertheless, available data from studies using different methodologies and designs are contradictory to the clinical results. The lack of evidence for clinical benefits could be explained by the absence of large randomized controlled trials and the fact that awake prone positioning sessions were much shorter than recommended prone positioning sessions in intubated ARDS patients.

Most of the complications described during prone placement in mechanically ventilated patients (airway obstruction, unplanned extubation, pressure ulcers, facial edema, and brachial plexus neuropathy) appear related to sedation and mechanical ventilation. Other complications such as transient oxygen desaturation and loss of venous access are described in awake pronation. Data are limited but published studies on prone positioning in the waking state have described no serious adverse events. However, some studies have reported little tolerance to prone-awake positioning sessions, with frequent side effects: musculoskeletal discomfort, nausea/vomiting, coughing or anxiety.

In addition to the length of a single prone positioning course, multiple short prone positioning sessions in the presence of trained and experienced personnel could be a solution to improve tolerance in awake patients and lead to clinical benefits [37]. The published data does not determine which patient's prone positioning may be beneficial or the best duration and frequency of prone positioning sessions.

Discussion

Prone positioning has been used in acute lung injury (ALI) / acute respiratory distress syndrome (ARDS) patients. Mechanical ventilation in the prone position, first documented in 1970, has been considered as a strategy for improving oxygenation and lung recruitment in acute respiratory failure. Mechanisms by which prone positioning may benefit patients with acute respiratory distress syndrome (ARDS) experiencing mechanical ventilation include enhanced ventilation-perfusion matching, increased expiratory lung volume, and prevention of ventilator-induced lung damage by more uniform diffusion of tidal volume through lung recruitment and alterations in chest wall mechanics.

Compared to the supine position (SP), placing the patients in PP results in a more uniform tidal volume allocation, partly changing the vertical pleural pressure gradient, which becomes more damaging in the dorsal regions. PP also enhances resting lung volume in the dorso-caudal areas by reducing overlapping pressure in both the heart and abdomen. On the other hand, pulmonary perfusion remains preferentially distributed to the dorsal lung regions, thus improving the general ventilation/alveolar perfusion relationships. The first studies have consistently shown better oxygenation. Although these studies did not demonstrate a mortality benefit from prone positioning, post hoc analysis of subgroups with more severe forms of respiratory insufficiency suggested a benefit. Early-onset of PP is possible to improve oxygenation than early-onset during the subacute phase.

The most consequential improvement in oxygenation occurs over a large period ranging from a few hours to several days. Meta-analyzes of randomized controlled trials indicate that PP furnishes a survival benefit only in patients with relatively severe ARDS (PaO_2 / FIO_2 10-12 h / session) [38]. The mixture of adjunct treatments (elevated PEEP, recruitment maneuvers, and inhaled vasodilators with PP) have an additive effect in enhancing oxygenation and may be especially useful in stabilizing gas exchange in very severe ARDS [39]. Awake prone positioning enhances oxygenation during prone positioning but perseverance after supination and impact on clinical outcomes remain undecided.

Due to its relative comfort of use and low side effects, prone positioning for non-intubated patients has been widely involved and examined in COVID-19 patients in both medical divisions and emergency rooms. Combination with NIV or HFNC is suggested to improve respiratory status benefits. Oxygen results are encouraging, but evidence of clinical outcomes, such as mortality or intubation rates Studies do not determine the best period and frequency of the prone positioning session and tolerance of prolonged prone positioning sessions is a problem. Many questions remain unanswered, and a systemic strategy is required. Multiple randomized trials, including a meta-trial, are ongoing to evaluate the clinical benefits of prone positioning in managing COVID patients. Shortly, prone-awake positioning could be a simple and inexpensive tool for managing hypoxemic IRA in spontaneously breathing, non-COVID and COVID patients.

Conclusion

Prone position is associated with reduced mortality in ARDS patients, as demonstrated by Guerin in 2013 and the Formal Guide to Treatment of ARDS suggested the use of PP for at least 16 h per day when P / F <150 (moderate - severe ARDS). A study in 20 healthy patients demonstrated end-tidal lung volume (LVEE) growth and respiratory rate reduction using HFNC indicated by electrical impedance tomography [3]. The etiology of ARDS reported by Ding et al. includes infectious disease in all cases, indicating that an early PP strategy with HFNC or NIV is safe and effective in patients with moderate ARDS and >95% SpO_2 in whom intubation it could be prevented [23].

Early application of PP with HFNC or NIV, specifically in patients with moderate non-intubated ARDS and with SpO_2> 95%, can avoid intubation. PP was normally well accepted, and the efficacy of the four supporting strategies on PaO_2 / FiO_2 was HFNC <HFNC + PP ≤ NIV <NIV + PP. Patients with severe ARDS were not suitable candidates for NFNC / NIV + PP, and the risk of complications with delayed intubation may be expanded. The results of the OPTIPRONE study on the use of PP in combination with HFNC in patients with ARDS with PaO_2 / FiO_2 <200 is expected. A prospective multi-center RCT is certified in the future in patients with moderate non-intubated ARDS to reach a firm conclusion.

References

[1] Mancebo J, Fernández R, Blanch L, Rialp G, Gordo F, Ferrer M, Rodríguez F, Garro P, Ricart P, Vallverdú I, Gich I, Castaño J, Saura P, Domínguez G, Bonet A, Albert RK. A multicenter trial of prolonged prone ventilation in severe acute respiratory distress syndrome. *Am J Respir Crit Care Med.* 2006 Jun 1;173(11): 1233-9. doi: 10.1164/rccm.200503-353OC. Epub 2006 Mar 23. PMID: 16556697.

[2] Bryan AC. Comments of a devil's advocate. *Am Rev Respir Dis.* 1974;110 (62):143-144.

[3] Guérin C, Reignier J, Richard JC, Beuret P, Gacouin A, Boulain T, Mercier E, Badet M, Mercat A, Baudin O, Clavel M, Chatellier D, Jaber S, Rosselli S, Mancebo J, Sirodot M, Hilbert G, Bengler C, Richecoeur J, Gainnier M, Bayle F, Bourdin G, Leray V, Girard R, Baboi L, Ayzac L; PROSEVA Study Group. Prone positioning in severe acute respiratory distress syndrome. *N Engl J Med.* 2013 Jun 6;368(23):2159-68. doi: 10.1056/NEJMoa1214103. Epub 2013 May 20. PMID: 23688302.

[4] Fan E, Del Sorbo L, Goligher EC, Hodgson CL, Munshi L, Walkey AJ, Adhikari NKJ, Amato MBP, Branson R, Brower RG, Ferguson ND, Gajic O, Gattinoni L, Hess D, Mancebo J, Meade MO, McAuley DF, Pesenti A, Ranieri VM, Rubenfeld GD, Rubin E, Seckel M, Slutsky AS, Talmor D, Thompson BT, Wunsch H, Uleryk E, Brozek J, Brochard LJ; American Thoracic Society, European Society of Intensive Care Medicine, and Society of Critical Care Medicine. An Official American Thoracic Society/European Society of Intensive Care Medicine/Society of Critical Care Medicine Clinical Practice Guideline: Mechanical Ventilation in Adult Patients with Acute Respiratory Distress Syndrome. Am J Respir Crit Care Med. 2017 May 1;195(9):1253-1263. doi: 10.1164/rccm.201703-0548ST. Erratum in: *Am J Respir Crit Care Med.* 2017 Jun 1;195(11):1540. PMID: 28459336.

[5] Zhou F, Yu T, Du R, Fan G, Liu Y, Liu Z, Xiang J, Wang Y, Song B, Gu X, Guan L, Wei Y, Li H, Wu X, Xu J, Tu S, Zhang Y, Chen H, Cao B. Clinical course and risk factors for mortality of adult inpatients with COVID-19 in Wuhan, China: a retrospective cohort study. *Lancet.* 2020 Mar 28;395(10229):1054-1062. doi: 10.1016/S0140-6736(20)30566-3. Epub 2020 Mar 11. Erratum in: Lancet. 2020 Mar 28;395(10229):1038. Erratum in: *Lancet.* 2020 Mar 28;395(10229):1038. PMID: 32171076; PMCID: PMC7270627.

[6] Sun Q, Qiu H, Huang M, Yang Y. Lower mortality of COVID-19 by early recognition and intervention: experience from Jiangsu Province. *Ann Intensive Care*. 2020 Mar 18;10(1):33. doi: 10.1186/s13613-020-00650-2. PMID: 32189136; PMCID: PMC7080931.

[7] Touchon F, Trigui Y, Prud'homme E, Lefebvre L, Giraud A, Dols AM, Martinez S, Bernardi M, Begne C, Granier P, Chanez P, Forel JM, Papazian L, Elharrar X. Awake prone positioning for hypoxaemic respiratory failure: past, COVID-19 and perspectives. *Eur Respir Rev*. 2021 May 5;30(160):210022. doi: 10.1183 /16000617.0022-2021. PMID: 33952601; PMCID: PMC8112009.

[8] Langer M, Mascheroni D, Marcolin R, Gattinoni L. The prone position in ARDS patients. A clinical study. *Chest*. 1988 Jul;94(1):103-7. doi: 10.1378/chest.94.1. 103. PMID: 3383620.

[9] Karbing DS, Panigada M, Bottino N, Spinelli E, Protti A, Rees SE, Gattinoni L. Changes in shunt, ventilation/perfusion mismatch, and lung aeration with PEEP in patients with ARDS: a prospective single-arm interventional study. *Crit Care*. 2020 Mar 23;24(1):111. doi: 10.1186/s13054-020-2834-6. PMID: 32293506; PMCID: PMC7092565.

[10] Gattinoni L, Pelosi P, Vitale G, Pesenti A, D'Andrea L, Mascheroni D. Body position changes redistribute lung computed-tomographic density in patients with acute respiratory failure. *Anesthesiology*. 1991 Jan;74(1):15-23. doi: 10.1097/ 00000542-199101000-00004. PMID: 1986640.

[11] Gattinoni L, Pesenti A, Carlesso E. Body position changes redistribute lung computed-tomographic density in patients with acute respiratory failure: impact and clinical fallout through the following 20 years. *Intensive Care Med*. 2013 Nov;39(11):1909-15. doi: 10.1007/s00134-013-3066-x. Epub 2013 Sep 12. PMID: 24026295.

[12] Kumaresan A, Gerber R, Mueller A, Loring SH, Talmor D. Effects of Prone Positioning on Transpulmonary Pressures and End-expiratory Volumes in Patients without Lung Disease. *Anesthesiology*. 2018 Jun;128(6):1187-1192. doi: 10.1097/ ALN.0000000000002159. PMID: 29521672.

[13] Pelosi P, Brazzi L, Gattinoni L. Prone position in acute respiratory distress syndrome. *Eur Respir J*. 2002 Oct;20(4):1017-28. doi: 10.1183/09031936. 02.00401702. PMID: 12412699.

[14] West JB, Dollery CT, Naimark A. Distribution of blood flow in isolated lung; relation to vascular and alveolar pressures. *J Appl Physiol* 1964; 19: 713–724.

[15] Slutsky AS, Ranieri VM. Ventilator-induced lung injury. *N Engl J Med* 2013; 369: 2126–2136.

[16] Cornejo RA, Díaz JC, Tobar EA, Bruhn AR, Ramos CA, González RA, Repetto CA, Romero CM, Gálvez LR, Llanos O, Arellano DH, Neira WR, Díaz GA, Zamorano AJ, Pereira GL. Effects of prone positioning on lung protection in patients with acute respiratory distress syndrome. *Am J Respir Crit Care Med*. 2013 Aug 15;188(4):440-8. doi: 10.1164/rccm.201207-1279OC. PMID: 23348974.

[17] Papazian L, Gainnier M, Marin V, Donati S, Arnal JM, Demory D, Roch A, Forel JM, Bongrand P, Brégeon F, Sainty JM. Comparison of prone positioning and high-frequency oscillatory ventilation in patients with acute respiratory distress

syndrome. *Crit Care Med*. 2005 Oct;33(10):2162-71. doi: 10.1097/01.ccm.0000181298.05474.2b. PMID: 16215365.

[18] Park MS, He Q, Edwards MG, Sergew A, Riches DW, Albert RK, Douglas IS. Mitogen-activated protein kinase phosphatase-1 modulates regional effects of injurious mechanical ventilation in rodent lungs. *Am J Respir Crit Care Med.* 2012 Jul 1;186(1):72-81. doi: 10.1164/rccm.201109-1593OC. Epub 2012 May 10. PMID: 22582160; PMCID: PMC3400991.

[19] Chaisupamongkollarp T, Preuthipan A, Vaicheeta S, Chantarojanasiri T, Kongvivekkajornkij W, Suwanjutha S. Prone position in spontaneously breathing infants with pneumonia. *Acta Paediatr*. 1999 Sep;88(9):1033-4. doi: 10.1080/08035259950168586. PMID: 10519350.

[20] Feltracco P, Serra E, Barbieri S, Milevoj M, Michieletto E, Carollo C, Rea F, Zanus G, Boetto R, Ori C. Non-invasive high-frequency percussive ventilation in the prone position after lung transplantation. *Transplant Proc*. 2012 Sep;44(7): 2016-21. doi: 10.1016/j.transproceed.2012.05.062. PMID: 22974896.

[21] Scaravilli V, Grasselli G, Castagna L, Zanella A, Isgrò S, Lucchini A, Patroniti N, Bellani G, Pesenti A. Prone positioning improves oxygenation in spontaneously breathing nonintubated patients with hypoxemic acute respiratory failure: A retrospective study. *J Crit Care*. 2015 Dec;30(6):1390-4. doi: 10.1016/j.jcrc.2015.07.008. Epub 2015 Jul 16. PMID: 26271685.

[22] Ding L, Wang L, Ma W, He H. Efficacy and safety of early prone positioning combined with HFNC or NIV in moderate to severe ARDS: a multi-center prospective cohort study. *Crit Care*. 2020 Jan 30;24(1):28. doi: 10.1186/s13054-020-2738-5. PMID: 32000806; PMCID: PMC6993481.

[23] https://www.formacionsanitaria.eu/documentos/Recomendations_WeVent.pdf. Last Accessed on 23/06/2020.

[24] Coppo A, Bellani G, Winterton D, Di Pierro M, Soria A, Faverio P, Cairo M, Mori S, Messinesi G, Contro E, Bonfanti P, Benini A, Valsecchi MG, Antolini L, Foti G. Feasibility and physiological effects of prone positioning in non-intubated patients with acute respiratory failure due to COVID-19 (PRON-COVID): a prospective cohort study. *Lancet Respir Med*. 2020 Aug;8(8):765-774. doi: 10.1016/S2213-2600(20)30268-X. Epub 2020 Jun 19. PMID: 32569585; PMCID: PMC7304954.

[25] Elharrar X, Trigui Y, Dols AM, Touchon F, Martinez S, Prud'homme E, Papazian L. Use of Prone Positioning in Nonintubated Patients With COVID-19 and Hypoxemic Acute Respiratory Failure. *JAMA*. 2020 Jun 9;323(22):2336-2338. doi: 10.1001/jama.2020.8255. PMID: 32412581; PMCID: PMC7229532.

[26] Despres C, Brunin Y, Berthier F, Pili-Floury S, Besch G. Prone positioning combined with high-flow nasal or conventional oxygen therapy in severe Covid-19 patients. *Crit Care*. 2020 May 26;24(1):256. doi: 10.1186/s13054-020-03001-6. PMID: 32456663; PMCID: PMC7250283.

[27] Ng Z, Tay WC, Ho CHB. Awake prone positioning for non-intubated oxygen dependent COVID-19 pneumonia patients. *Eur Respir J*. 2020 Jul 23;56(1): 2001198. doi: 10.1183/13993003.01198-2020. PMID: 32457195; PMCID: PMC7251246.

[28] Pb S, Mittal S, Madan K, Mohan A, Tiwari P, Hadda V, Pandey RM, Guleria R. Awake prone positioning in non-intubated patients for the management of hypoxemia in COVID-19: A systematic review and meta-analysis. *Monaldi Arch Chest Dis.* 2021 Apr 22;91(2). doi: 10.4081/monaldi.2021.1623. PMID: 33926179.

[29] Sartini C, Tresoldi M, Scarpellini P, Tettamanti A, Carcò F, Landoni G, Zangrillo A. Respiratory Parameters in Patients With COVID-19 After Using Non-invasive Ventilation in the Prone Position Outside the Intensive Care Unit. *JAMA*. 2020 Jun 9;323(22):2338-2340. doi: 10.1001/jama.2020.7861. PMID: 32412606; PMCID: PMC7229533.

[30] Chiumello D, Chiodaroli E, Coppola S, Cappio Borlino S, Granata C, Pitimada M, Wendel Garcia PD. Awake prone position reduces work of breathing in patients with COVID-19 ARDS supported by CPAP. *Ann Intensive Care.* 2021 Dec 20;11(1):179. doi: 10.1186/s13613-021-00967-6. PMID: 34928455; PMCID: PMC8686083.

[31] Caputo ND, Strayer RJ, Levitan R. Early Self-Proning in Awake, Non-intubated Patients in the Emergency Department: A Single ED's Experience During the COVID-19 Pandemic. *Acad Emerg Med.* 2020 May;27(5):375-378. doi: 10.1111/acem.13994. PMID: 32320506; PMCID: PMC7264594.

[32] Thompson AE, Ranard BL, Wei Y, Jelic S. Prone Positioning in Awake, Nonintubated Patients With COVID-19 Hypoxemic Respiratory Failure. *JAMA Intern Med.* 2020 Nov 1;180(11):1537-1539. doi: 10.1001/jamainternmed. 2020.3030. PMID: 32584946; PMCID: PMC7301298.

[33] Hallifax RJ, Porter BM, Elder PJ, Evans SB, Turnbull CD, Hynes G, Lardner R, Archer K, Bettinson HV, Nickol AH, Flight WG, Chapman SJ, Hardinge M, Hoyles RK, Saunders P, Sykes A, Wrightson JM, Moore A, Ho LP, Fraser E, Pavord ID, Talbot NP, Bafadhel M, Petousi N, Rahman NM; Oxford Respiratory Group. Successful awake proning is associated with improved clinical outcomes in patients with COVID-19: single-centre high-dependency unit experience. *BMJ Open Respir Res.* 2020 Sep;7(1):e000678. doi: 10.1136/bmjresp-2020-000678. PMID: 32928787; PMCID: PMC7490910.

[34] Padrão EMH, Valente FS, Besen BAMP, Rahhal H, Mesquita PS, de Alencar JCG, da Costa MGP, Wanderley APB, Emerenciano DL, Bortoleto FM, Fortes JCL, Marques B, de Souza SFB, Marchini JFM, Neto RAB, de Souza HP; COVIDTEAM. Awake Prone Positioning in COVID-19 Hypoxemic Respiratory Failure: Exploratory Findings in a Single-center Retrospective Cohort Study. *Acad Emerg Med.* 2020 Dec;27(12):1249-1259. doi: 10.1111/acem.14160. Epub 2020 Nov 21. PMID: 33107664.

[35] Ferrando C, Mellado-Artigas R, Gea A, Arruti E, Aldecoa C, Adalia R, Ramasco F, Monedero P, Maseda E, Tamayo G, Hernández-Sanz ML, Mercadal J, Martín-Grande A, Kacmarek RM, Villar J, Suárez-Sipmann F; COVID-19 Spanish ICU Network. Awake prone positioning does not reduce the risk of intubation in COVID-19 treated with high-flow nasal oxygen therapy: a multicenter, adjusted cohort study. *Crit Care.* 2020 Oct 6;24(1):597. doi: 10.1186/s13054-020-03314-6. PMID: 33023669; PMCID: PMC7537953.

[36] Telias I, Katira BH, Brochard L. Is the Prone Position Helpful During Spontaneous Breathing in Patients With COVID-19? *JAMA*. 2020 Jun 9;323(22):2265-2267. doi: 10.1001/jama.2020.8539. PMID: 32412579.

[37] Munshi L, Del Sorbo L, Adhikari NKJ, Hodgson CL, Wunsch H, Meade MO, Uleryk E, Mancebo J, Pesenti A, Ranieri VM, Fan E. Prone Position for Acute Respiratory Distress Syndrome. A Systematic Review and Meta-Analysis. *Ann Am Thorac Soc*. 2017 Oct;14(Supplement_4):S280-S288. doi: 10.1513/AnnalsATS.201704-343OT. PMID: 29068269.

[38] Park SY, Kim HJ, Yoo KH, Park YB, Kim SW, Lee SJ, Kim EK, Kim JH, Kim YH, Moon JY, Min KH, Park SS, Lee J, Lee CH, Park J, Byun MK, Lee SW, Rlee C, Jung JY, Sim YS. The efficacy and safety of prone positioning in adults patients with acute respiratory distress syndrome: a meta-analysis of randomized controlled trials. *J Thorac Dis.* 2015 Mar;7(3):356-67. doi: 10.3978/j.issn.2072-1439.2014.12.49. PMID: 25922713; PMCID: PMC4387391.

[39] Das A, Haque M, Chikhani M, Cole O, Wang W, Hardman JG, Bates DG. Hemodynamic effects of lung recruitment maneuvers in acute respiratory distress syndrome. *BMC Pulm Med*. 2017 Feb 8;17(1):34. doi: 10.1186/s12890-017-0369-7. PMID: 28178996; PMCID: PMC5299789.

Chapter 6

Exacerbation in Patients with Nasal Cannula Oxygen Therapy

Héctor Molina Corona[1,*], MD
and Vanessa Alejandra Villarreal Vargas[2], MD

[1] Pulmonology Department, Hospital General Fray Junípero Serra,
Institute of Security and Social Services for State Workers, Tijuana, B.C., México
[2] Audiology Department,
Tijuana Center for the Deaf and Hearing, Tijuana, B.C. México

Abstract

Chronic obstructive pulmonary disease (COPD) is a quite common disease, dynamic and heterogenous. Through the years, this disease has had many changes, in its definition, classification and treatment options. In the recent 2022 report of the Global Initiative for Chronic Obstructive Lung Disease (GOLD) there are new proposals for its classification, adding the terms early COPD, mild COPD, COPD in young people (age range from 20-50 years old) and Pre-COPD [1]. In the near future this will impact the disease concerning therapy options.

Acute exacerbation of COPD (AECOPD) is frequently associated to hypercapnic respiratory failure (HRF) and classically the main therapeutic option was invasive mechanical ventilation (IMV), until recent years that non-invasive ventilation (NIV) has been available with satisfactory results. Also, high flow nasal cannula oxygen therapy (HFNC) is a valuable tool in treatment of AECOPD with HRF, as shown in many studies. Conventional oxygen therapy (COT) is still a useful tool in this area, with its limitations. The main goal of this chapter was to

* Corresponding Author's Email: neumohecx@hotmail.com.

In: Nasal High Flow and Non-Invasive Ventilatory Support
Editors: A. M. Esquinas, D. A. Lagonidis, P. Silva Santos et al.
ISBN: 979-8-88697-420-1

review recently available data and to propose a basis for adequate escalation therapy.

Keywords: chronic obstructive pulmonary disease, non-invasive ventilation, hypercapnic respiratory failure, high-flow nasal cannula oxygen therapy

Introduction

Chronic obstructive pulmonary disease (COPD) is a common, preventable, and treatable disease characterized by persistent respiratory symptoms and airflow limitation due to airway and/or alveolar abnormalities. Prevalence is variable, depending on the region. In the Latin American Project for the Investigation of Obstructive Lung Disease (PLATINO), its prevalence was estimated as low as 7.8% in Mexico City and high as 19.7% in Montevideo, Uruguay. It is associated to great socioeconomic burden due to disability [1]. In a recent report by the World Health Association (WHO) it is the third leading cause of death worldwide, around 3.2 million deaths were registered in 2019 [1, 2].

Exacerbation is considered an acute worsening of respiratory symptoms that require additional treatment [1, 2]. Respiratory therapy is a particularly valuable tool for the treatment of acute exacerbation, from oxygen therapy and high flow nasal cannula to non-invasive ventilation. Which is the best method for an acute exacerbation of COPD? When to apply them? Escalation proposal? The focus of this chapter is on oxygen therapy, high flow nasal cannula and non-invasive ventilation based on recent data.

Acute Exacerbations of COPD

AECOPD is associated with increased inflammation of the airway, hyperinflation and increased mucous production, contributing to augmented symptoms such as dyspnea, increased cough, increased sputum purulence and wheezing. Exacerbations of COPD are significant, due to negative impact in health status and progression of the disease, resulting in limitation of working days. It is known that within the three years of detection of COPD, over 70% of patients will have an AECOPD and up to 47% may have two or more events regardless of airflow severity.

There are many risk factors and triggers associated to AECOPD such as tobacco smoking, air pollution, severe airflow limitation, bronchiectasis, infections mainly of virus origin and some bacteria, blood eosinophil count, and prior exacerbations and comorbidities (hyperglycaemia, hypertension, atherosclerosis). AECOPD requires hospitalization, about 20% of these patients present or develop hypercapnic respiratory failure (HRF), which is an indicator for increased risk of death. When respiratory acidosis is present, respiratory muscles fail in achieving adequate alveolar ventilation despite of diaphragmatic activity. Hyperinflation also contributes to respiratory muscle compromise. As the capacity of the respiratory pump exceeds, rapid shallow breathing develops with increased respiratory rate and small tidal volumes, leading to respiratory acidosis [3].

Treatment of exacerbation is focused on control of symptoms with bronchodilators, steroids (inhaled and systemic), antibiotics, oxygen therapy, non-invasive ventilation, and invasive ventilation [3]. Considering the impact of AECOPD on the disease itself, there are some recent prediction models available. One the most recently reported is a digital application called COPD-Predict-TM by Patel *et al.* in a 6-month prospective observational study of 90 patients with frequent COPD exacerbations. This system showed a high sensitivity of 97.9% which indicates that if there is an exacerbation patients and healthcare team are informed accurately; it provides safe, personalised, and preventative care for patients with COPD [4]. Yii *et al.* developed a model that focuses on assessing the risk of hospitalization of COPD exacerbations using treatable traits and history of exacerbations. Presenting excellent concurrence between predicted and observed annual hospitalized exacerbation rates (AUC of 0.789 indicating good discriminative accuracy, significantly higher than the Global Initiative for Chronic Obstructive Lung Disease (GOLD) risk assessment criterion [5].

Oxygen Therapy

Oxygen therapy is generally used during acute respiratory failure. This is also the case for acute exacerbation of COPD when oxygen desaturation is detected, and hypoxemia is confirmed. Along years of research, it is well known that patients with COPD during acute exacerbation, are at risk of developing hypercapnic respiratory failure (HRF) [6]. When a patient starts receiving oxygen, blood gases must be measured to ensure adequate therapy without carbon dioxide retention. Some patients have recurrent episodes of

HRF during exacerbations. It has been shown that there is higher risk when hyperoxemia with PaO_2 above 75 mmHg is present.

However, it is difficult to predict which patients will develop HRF in response to oxygen therapy, so it is important to draw arterial blood gas (ABG) sample promptly during an AECOPD. It is recommended to maintain SaO_2 levels at a target of 88-92% during AECOPD and the use of oxygen using a Venturi mask with a fraction of inspired oxygen (FiO_2) of 24% at 2-3 Litres/min or nasal cannula at 1-2 Litres/min or FiO_2 of 28% Venturi mask at 4 Litres/min, while the result of ABG sample is available to discard or confirm respiratory acidosis. When HRF is discarded, the suggested aim for SaO_2 is of 94-98%, apart from patients with previous HRF with use of non-invasive ventilation (target SaO_2 88-92%) in which case NIV should be started promptly [6].

High-Flow Nasal Cannula Oxygen

High-flow nasal cannula oxygen (HFNC) is a therapy that has been available since early 2000's. It has been used with remarkable success in the treatment of acute respiratory failure (ARF) and in recent years as a tool for HRF in AECOPD. Using a nasal cannula with a single heated circuit connected to an air/oxygen blender and active heating humidifier; administers oxygen with high flow from 20 to 60 Litres/min and fraction of oxygen (FiO_2) as high as 100%. This device has an open system it does not facilitate tidal volume (Vt) and minute ventilation.

There are many known effects of HFNC:

1) Provides heated (37°C) and humidified air-oxygen admixture. Delivery of adequately conditioned gas to patients is possible. It reduces inflammatory response associated to dry and cold gases, avoiding ciliary injury and keeps the water content of the bronchial secretions consistent.
2) Washing out of carbon dioxide of the pharyngeal dead space. It is the only non-invasive respiratory support that doesn't increase dead space [7, 8],
3) Generates considerable Positive end of expiration pressure (PEEP) of pharyngeal dead space (up to 8cm$H_2$0). As shown in many studies, pressure increases as flow increases.

4) Guarantees a more stable fraction of inspired oxygen (FiO_2); during HFNC actual FiO_2 is close to predicted FiO_2 [7,8]. HFNC offers more comfort to the patient as compared to conventional oxygen therapy and NIV.

A systematic review of literature of HFNC in AECOPD, showed minimal differences in gas exchange ($PaCO_2$ and PaO_2), respiratory rate and clinical outcomes such as intubation rate, 28-30- day mortality, ICU length of stay [8]. A group in Argentina proposed the use of HFNC oxygen with high velocity nasal insufflation (HVNI) as a first-line ventilation support in COPD patients with acute HRF.

It was multicentre prospective analytic observational pilot study with forty subjects with severe COPD and HRF in the ICU. HFNC oxygen with high velocity nasal insufflation was used, which was effective for reducing respiratory rate to a 27% after and significant $PaCO_2$ reduction after one hour, with 18% failure (comparable to NIV); further investigation is needed with RCT [9].

Non-Invasive Ventilation

Invasive mechanical ventilation (IMV) for many years, was the mainstay treatment for AECOPD with AHRF nonresponsive to conventional therapy (bronchodilators, corticosteroids, and oxygen therapy), with successful reversal of hypercapnia. However, IMV is associated to significant risks of morbidity (ventilation associated pneumonia, prolonged hospitalization and long ICU stay), mortality and difficult weaning. In the last 25 years or more, NIV has proven to be an alternative, but still is underused because of some concerns related to outcomes [10, 11, 12].

It is well known that positive pressure ventilation unloads fatigued ventilatory muscles. With different interfaces used (nasal, oronasal, full face), it offers short intermittent periods of ventilation, interaction of the patient (talking, eating), lack of sedation and the opportunity of involvement of the patient in therapeutic decisions [10, 11, 12]. Many randomized controlled trials (RCTs) meta-analyses and case series with AECOPD have demonstrated the efficacy of NIV. It has been used to prevent development of acute respiratory acidosis (normal or raised $PaCO_2$, normal pH); to prevent use of invasive mechanical ventilation (IMV) in mild to moderate acute respiratory acidosis (pH 7.25- 7.35) with respiratory distress ($PaCO_2$>45) and as an alternative to IMV in patients with severe acidosis (pH<7.25) and very severe respiratory distress [10, 11, 12].

The review of 17 RCTs of AECOPD with ARF by Osadnik *et al.* (Cochrane Database 2017) reported that NIV decreased the risk of mortality (by almost half), need for invasive mechanical ventilation (IMV) following endotracheal intubation (ETI) (by 65%), length of Stay (LOS) in hospital (by almost 3 and half days), incidence of complications (other than those related to NIV), reduces mortality by 46%. NIV also leads to improvement in biochemical parameters, within an hour, an increase in pH (by 0.05), oxygenation (by 7.47 mmHg) and a reduction in carbon dioxide (by 4.62 mmHg) are often achieved [10, 11, 12]. NIV in AECOPD with ARF with no or very mild acidosis ($PaCO_2$ >=45 mmHg, pH> 7.35) in some studies was not beneficial. In patients without acidosis, comparing use of NIV plus standard therapy versus standard treatment alone showed poor tolerance of NIV and no benefit of use of NIV [10-12].

Initiation of NIV should involve a team with expertise, detailed knowledge of several factors that include the timing of initiation, magnitude of treatment effect and likelihood of successful treatment. Because of the need of a predictive model to improve the decision regarding ventilation, Hartley et al. developed a model the Non-invasive Ventilation Outcomes (NIVO) score. By using simple, readily available information applicable to the real world, it allows accurate risk stratification of patients admitted to hospital with AECOPD with acidosis and AHRF that required assisted ventilation [11,12, 13].

Conclusion

COT is useful in acute respiratory failure during AECOPD, although attention must be taken concerning hypercapnia as hyperoxemia can worsen this condition. When respiratory acidosis is present and/or respiratory deterioration, escalation from COT to HFNC or NIV. Many studies have evaluated differences between HFNC and NIV. They both have beneficial effects in reducing $PaCO_2$ and in unloading respiratory muscles.

Many studies have evaluated differences between HFNC and NIV. In the study by Cortegiani *et al.* HFNC demonstrated a statistically non-inferior effect on reducing $PaCO_2$ during the first two hours, followed by the need of NIV in 32% of patients after 6 hours of therapy [14]. The observational cohort study by Sun et al, showed no significant differences in respiratory rate,

$PaCO_2$, and PaO_2/FiO_2 ratio 24 hrs after treatment between HFNC and NIV. As well as total days of respiratory support, ICU, or hospital total length of stay. However, intolerance was more frequent with NIV due to nasal skin breakdown (20.9%) [15]. The decision of escalation starting with COT to HFNC and NIV, also depends on availability of equipment and staff experience.

For AECOPD with HRF, we think it is reasonable to start with a trial of either HFNC or NIV for one to two hours. If stable, we recommend persisting course of treatment. If deterioration is present (worsening of respiratory distress and/or respiratory acidosis) IMV must be started without delay, thinking on safety first for the patient. However, if HFNC failed, NIV can be the next step, if the patient can cooperate and considering clinical conditions (e.g., need of vasopressors, need of ICU) and level of respiratory acidosis/hypercapnia; we recommend a trial of 30-40 minutes with clinical and blood gas analysis to re-evaluate the next step.

References

[1] Global Initiative for Chronic Obstructive Lung Disease (GOLD). *Global Strategy for the management and prevention of chronic obstructive lung disease*. 2021 REPORT.

[2] World Health Organization (WHO) webpage, www.who.int, Newsroom *Chronic Obstructive Pulmonary Disease*, June 21, 2021.

[3] Viniol C, Vogelmeir CF. Exacerbations of COPD. *European Respiratory Review*, 2018; 27: 1-9.

[4] Patel N, Kinmond K, Jones P, Birks P, Spiteri MA. Validation of COPDPredict TM: Unique combination of remote monitoring and exacerbation prediction to support Preventative management of COPD exacerbations. *International Journal of Chronic Obstructive Pulmonary Disease,* 2021. 16, 1887-1899. Dovepress.

[5] Yii A, Loh CH, Tiew PY, Xu H, Taha A, Koh J, Tan J, Lapperre TS, Anzueto A, Tee A KH. A clinical prediction model for hospitalized COPD exacerbations based on "treatable traits." *International Journal of Chronic Obstructive Pulmonary Disease,* 2019: 14, 719-728. Dovepress.

[6] Guideline for Oxygen Use in Adults in Healthcare and Emergency Settings. British Thoracic Society Emergency Oxygen Guideline Development Group. *THORAX,* Volume 72, Supplement1. June 2017.

[7] Nishimura N. High-Flow Nasal Cannula Oxygen Therapy in Adults: Physiological Benefits, Indication, Clinical Benefits, and Adverse effects. *Respiratory Care*, April 2016; 61(4): 529-541.

[8] Pisani L, Astuto M, Prediletto I, Longhini F. High Flow through nasal cannula in exacerbated COPD patients: A systematic review. *Pulmonology,* 2019; 25 (6):348-354.

[9] Plotnikow GA, Acocce M, Fredes S, Tiribelli N, Setten M, Dorado J, Guaymas M. Ilutovich S, Rodriguez PO, Cesio CE, Scapellato JL, Vasquez DN. High Flow Oxygen Therapy Application in Chronic Obstructive Pulmonary Disease Patients with Acute Hypercapnic Respiratory Failure: A Multicentre Study. *Critical Care Explorations Journal*, February 2021, Volume 3, Number 2: 1-8.

[10] Rochwerg B, Brochard L, Elliott MW, Hess D, Hill NS, Nava S, Navalesi P (members of the steering committee); Antonelli M, Brozek J, Conti G, Ferrer M, Guntupalli K, Jaber S, Keenan S, Mancebo J, Mehta S, Raoof S (members of the task force). Official ERS/ATS clinical practice guidelines: Non-invasive ventilation for acute respiratory failure. *Eur Respir J,* 2017; 50: 1602426.

[11] Chawla R, Dixit SB, Zirpe KG, Chaudhry D, Khilnani GC, Mehta Y, Khatib KI, Jagiasi BG, Chanchalani G, Mishra RC, Samavedam S, Govil D, Gupta S, Prayag S, Rmasubban S, Dobariya J, Mrwah V, Sehgal I, Jog SA, Kulkarni AP. ISCCM Guidelines for the Use of Non-invasive Ventilation in Acute Respiratory Failure in Adult ICUs. *Indian J Crit Care Med,* 2020; 24(Suppl 1): S61–S81.

[12] Hartley T, Lane ND, Steer J, Elliott MW, Sovani MP, Curtis HJ, Fuller ER, Murphy PB, Shrikrishna D, Lewis KE, Ward NR, Turnbull CD, Hart N, Bourke SC. The NIV Outcomes (NIVO) Score: prediction of in-hospital mortality in exacerbations of COPD requiring assisted ventilation. *Eur Respir J*, 2021; in press. https://doi.org/10.1183/13993003.04042-2020.

[13] Osadnik CR, Tee VS, Carson-Chahhoud KV, Picot J, Wedzicha JA, Smith BJ. Non-invasive ventilation for the management of acute hypercapnic respiratory failure due to exacerbation of chronic obstructive pulmonary disease. *Cochrane Database of Systematic Reviews*, 2017, Issue 7. Art. No.: CD004104.

[14] Cortegiani A, Longhini F, Madotto F, Groff P, Scala R, Crimi C, Carlucci A, Bruni A, Garofalo E, Raineri SM, Tonelli R, Comellini V, Lupia E, Vetrugno L, Clini E, Giarratano A, Nava S, Navalesi P, Gregoretti C and the HF.-AECOPD study investigators. Research Open Access: High flow nasal therapy versus non-invasive ventilation as initial ventilatory strategy in COPD exacerbation: A multicentre non-inferiority randomized trial. *Critical Care*, 2020. 24:692: 1-13.BMC.

[15] Sun J, Li Y, Ling B, Zhu Q, Hu Y, Tan D, Geng P, Xu J. High flow nasal cannula oxygen therapy versus non-invasive ventilation for chronic obstructive pulmonary disease with acute-moderate hypercapnic respiratory failure: an observational cohort study International *Journal of Chronic Obstructive Pulmonary Disease,* 2019:14; 1229-1237.

Chapter 7

Domiciliary Use of High-Flow Nasal Cannula Oxygen Therapy

Margarida Matias*, **MD**
Pulmonology Department, West Lisbon Hospital Center, Lisboa, Portugal

Abstract

High-flow nasal cannula (HFNC) was developed for acute hypoxemic respiratory failure; however, it is becoming an upcoming treatment for several situations. Recent studies suggest that HFNC may have a role in Chronic obstructive pulmonary disease (COPD) patients either hypoxemic or with global respiratory failure intolerant to conventional therapies. However, HFNC as a long-term use in stable hypercapnic COPD patients rises some concerns about the possibility of CO_2 retention, which according to the literature does not happen.

In patients with chronic mucus hypersecretion, such as chronic bronchitis, bronchiectasis, and cystic fibrosis, HNFC improves lung clearance. The clinical applications of HFNC in interstitial lung disease and for palliative care have also been a subject of research. The physiological effects of HFNC, combined with its simplicity and comfortability, make HFNC an ideal candidate for long-term use though more evidence is needed to incorporate HNFC in standard clinical practice. In this chapter we will discuss different situations and pathologies in which HFNC can have a domiciliary use.

Keywords: high-flow nasal cannula, chronic obstructive pulmonary disease, chronic respiratory failure

* Corresponding Author's Email: margaridavmatias@gmail.com.

In: Nasal High Flow and Non-Invasive Ventilatory Support
Editors: A. M. Esquinas, D. A. Lagonidis, P. Silva Santos et al.
ISBN: 979-8-88697-420-1

Introduction

High-flow nasal cannula (HFNC) was primarily developed for management of apnea in premature neonate. In adults it was established in acute and critical care settings for treating mild-to-moderate acute hypoxic failure and ventilator weaning. However, the indications for HFNC have been expanding [1, 2].

In the last years the development of simpler HFNC devices, suitable for domiciliary use, allied to the comfort referred by patients and its physiological effects, has provided a new opportunity for respiratory support in several clinical respiratory conditions such as stable chronic obstructive pulmonary disease (COPD), during rehabilitation or for domiciliary palliative care [3].

Long-Term Use of NHFT in Stable COPD Patients

In patients with COPD and chronic respiratory failure, long-term oxygen therapy (LTOT) and non-invasive mechanical ventilation (NIMV) have been the therapeutic choices with specific criteria.[4] These respiratory supports may be poorly tolerated by some patients, NIMV in some patients is inapplicable due to discomfort associated with facial and nasal interface, high pressure intolerance, difficulty in synchronising breathing, claustrophobia and abdominal distension; LTOT compliance may be suboptimal [5, 6].

Recent studies suggest that HFNC may have a place in selected cases of COPD patients, either hypoxemic or with global respiratory failure, where its use is yet not well studied and still controversial [5, 7].

Hypercapnic Respiratory Failure

Several mechanisms have been advocated to explain the effect of HFNC. HFNC provides a continuous high flow that reduces the anatomical dead space in the upper airways, allowing a higher fraction of minute ventilation to participate in gas exchange and subsequentially $PaCO_2$ washout, even with reduction in respiratory rate [5]. The delivered flow is much higher than the patient spontaneous inspiratory flow, so actual FiO_2 is close to the predicted one and the exhaled air in the upper airways is replaced uninterruptedly by fresh air with low CO_2, leading to less CO_2 rebreathing [5, 6]. It also induces an increase in airway pressure, no more than 3 cmH_2O [8] which goes against intrinsic positive end-expiratory pressure and may also allow the removal of CO2 and reduce respiratory effort.

HFNC has other benefits due to humidification and heating of the inspired air: attenuation of inspiratory resistance, increased mucociliary function, and provides greater comfort, when compared to traditional oxygenation devices and better quality of life [2, 5, 9]. Therefore, it provides better comfort, compared with NMV, and a more efficient oxygenation than LTOT [5, 7].

For all the above HFNC seems to be an alternative to NMV for chronic hypercapnic COPD patients. Although major variation exists in COPD patients included in the trials and HFNC settings used therefore the evidence is still limited.

Hypoxemic Respiratory Failure

As expected, and far less controversially, HFNC has a role on patients with COPD and chronic hypoxic failure. In these population, with two or more exacerbations in the preceding year, HFNC significantly reduced acute exacerbations by about 40%, reduces hospital admissions, and symptoms, but without any effect on all-causes mortality [10]. It has been speculated that the reduction of exacerbations is likely because of humidification on airway clearance.

Based on available evidence, to hypoxemic patients with recurrent exacerbations and chronic hypercapnic patients it was suggested the following parameters of HFNC: flow 20-30L/min, FiO_2 based on peripherical saturation of O_2, and a 37ºC temperature [6].

Exercise Capacity

HNFC increases exercise capacity for stable COPD patients, they were able to improve the duration of exercise with less symptoms, better oxygenation and better breathing pattern compared with low-flow oxygen delivery [5].

Further Investigation

Although there is a rationale for using HFNC in COPD patients even in stable condition, its use is still limited and the impact on long-term outcomes has yet to be described [5]. Further studies are needed in well-defined patients' groups to assess optimal parameters of HFNC, effectiveness of domiciliary HFNC as a replacement to LTOT in hypoxemic patients, as an add-on to LTOT or as an alternative to NIMV in chronic hypercapnic COPD patients. Cost-effectiveness of HFNC is still uncertain.

Elshof et al., suggest research focus on hypoxemic COPD patients who exacerbate frequently to assess the potential clinical impact on admission reduction and a randomized control trial for hypercapnic to show whether HFNC is an alternative to NIMV in reducing hypercapnia and improvement in patient-related outcomes [6].

More evidence is therefore needed to incorporate NHFT in standard clinical practice.

Management of Chronic Mucus Hypersecretion

Chronic conditions such as chronic bronchitis, bronchiectasis and cystic fibrosis are associated with a persistent increase in mucus secretion, Hasani et al., reported that HNFC at 37°C for 3h/day for 6 days, significantly improved lung clearance in these pathologies [11]. In cystic fibrosis may have combined advantages improving both ventilation by reducing the work of breathing and airway clearance. In patients with bronchiectasis and COPD also reduces the number of days to exacerbation, increases time to the first exacerbation and reduces frequency of exacerbations (2.97/patient/year vs. 3.63/patient/year) compared to the standard therapy [12]. The benefits of HFNC in patients with these conditions deserve further investigation.

Interstitial Lung Disease

The clinical applications of HFNC in interstitial lung disease (ILD) patients are subject of research. Bräunlich et al., verified a PEEP effect in IPF patients associated with reduced respiratory rate. HFNC may have a role for end-stage ILD patients with severe hypoxemia, as palliative treatment [13].

Palliative Care

The use of HFNC has been extended to the palliative care, although there have been a limited number of reports mostly due to issues with oxygen supplies [14]. Studies in patients with end-stage respiratory failure, including interstitial lung diseases, COPD and cancer, showed a poor survival but HFNC allowed patients to return home and to be treated at reasonable cost. The role of this device for palliative care needs further consideration [15].

Conclusion

HFNC appears to be a safe, viable and highly promising alternative for patients with COPD intolerant to NIMV as a long-term treatment and may become a reality in standard clinical practice.

Retention of CO_2 does not seem to occur with the use of HFNC in hypercapnic patients.

In hypoxemic patients with recurrent exacerbations, HFNC reduces acute exacerbations and hospital admissions. In patients with a persistent increase in mucus secretion HNFC improves lung clearance. HFNC use is still limited and its impact on long-term outcomes has yet to be described.

References

[1] Frat J-P, Thille A W, Mercat A, Girault C, Ragot S, Perbet S, Prat G, Boulain T, Morawiec, E, Cottereau A, Devaquet J, Nseir S. High-Flow Oxygen through Nasal Cannula in Acute Hypoxemic Respiratory Failure. *N. Engl. J. Med.* 2015;372(23): 2185-2196. doi:10.1056/nejmoa1503326.

[2] Papazian L, Corley A, Hess D, Fraser J F, Frat J P, Guitton C, Jaber S, Maggiore S M, Nava S, Rello J, Ricard J D, Stephan F, Trisolini R and Azoulay E. Use of high-flow nasal cannula oxygenation in ICU adults: a narrative review. *Intensive Care Med.* 2016;42(9):1336-1349. doi:10.1007/s00134-016-4277-8.

[3] Schisano L S and M. High-flow nasal cannula oxygen therapy as an emerging option for respiratory failure: the present and the future. *Ther. Adv. Vaccines.* 2018;9(6): 259-261. doi:10.1177/https.

[4] Ergan B, Oczkowski S, Rochwerg B, Carlucci A, Chatwin M, Clini E, Elliott M, Gonzalez-Bermejo J, Hart N, Lujan M, Nasilowski J, Nava S, Pepin J L, Pisani L, Storre J H, Wijkstra P, Tonia T, Boyd J, Scala R, Windisch W. European Respiratory Society guidelines on long-term home non-invasive ventilation for management of COPD. *Eur. Respir. J.* 2019;54(3). doi:10.1183/13993003.01003-2019.

[5] Pisani L, Vega M L. Use of Nasal High Flow in Stable COPD: Rationale and Physiology. *COPD J. Chronic Obstr. Pulm. Dis.* 2017;14(3):346-350. doi:10.1080/15412555.2017.1315715.

[6] Elshof J, Duiverman M L. Clinical Evidence of Nasal High-Flow Therapy in Chronic Obstructive Pulmonary Disease Patients. *Respiration*. 2020;99(2):140-153. doi:10.1159/000505583.

[7] Pisani L, Fasano L, Corcione N, Comellini V, Musti MA, Brandao M, Bottone D Calderini E, Navalesi P, Nava S. Change in pulmonary mechanics and the effect on breathing pattern of high flow oxygen therapy in stable hypercapnic COPD. *Thorax*. 2017;72(4):373-375. doi:10.1136/thoraxjnl-2016-209673.

[8] Parke R, McGuinness S, Eccleston M. Nasal high-flow therapy delivers low level positive airway pressure. *Br. J. Anaesth*. 2009;103(6):886-890. doi:10.1093/bja/aep 280.

[9] Nagata K, Kikuchi T, Horie T, Shiraki A, KitajimaT, KadowakiT, Tokioka F, Chohnabayashi N, Watanabe A, Sato S, Tomii K. Domiciliary high-flow nasal cannula oxygen therapy for patients with stable hypercapnic chronic obstructive pulmonary disease a multicenter randomized crossover trial. *Ann. Am. Thorac. Soc*. 2018;15(4):432-439. doi:10.1513/AnnalsATS.201706-425OC.

[10] Storgaard L H, Hockey H U, Laursen B S, Weinreich U M. Long-term effects of oxygen-enriched high-flow nasal cannula treatment in copd patients with chronic hypoxemic respiratory failure. *Int. J. COPD*. 2018;13:1195-1205. doi:10.2147/ COPD.S159666.

[11] Hasani A, Chapman T H, McCool D, Smith R E, Dilworth J P, Agnew J E. Domiciliary humidification improves lung mucociliary clearance in patients with bronchiectasis. *Chron. Respir. Dis*. 2008;5(2):81-86. doi:10.1177/147997230708 7190.

[12] Rea H, McAuley S, Jayaram L, Garrett J, Hockey H, Storey L, O'Donnell G, Haru L, Payton M, O'Donnell K. The clinical utility of long-term humidification therapy in chronic airway disease. *Respir Med*. 2010;104(4):525-533. doi:10.1016/j.rmed. 2009.12.016.

[13] Bräunlich J, Beyer D, Mai D, Hammerschmidt S, Seyfarth H J, Wirtz H. Effects of nasal high flow on ventilation in volunteers, COPD and idiopathic pulmonary fibrosis patients. *Respiration*. 2013;85(4):319-325. doi:10.1159/000342027.

[14] Goda K, Kenzaka T, Kuriyama K, Hoshijima M, Akita H. End-of-life home care of an interstitial pneumonia patient supported by high-flow nasal cannula therapy: A case report. *World J. Clin. Cases*. 2020;8(20):4853-4857. doi:10.12998/wjcc.v8. i20.4853.

[15] Dolydon. Characteristics and outcome of patients set up on high-flow oxygen therapy at home. *Ther. Adv. Vaccines*. 2018;9(6):259-261. doi:10.1177/https.

Chapter 8

Support during Exercise in Chronic Obstructive Pulmonary Disease

Jonathan Cámara Fernandez*, MD
Pulmonology Service, Sant Joan de Deu Health Park, Barcelona, Spain

Abstract

High-flow nasal cannula therapy represents a new form of non-invasive therapy for patients with hypoxemic and hypercapnic respiratory failure. Thermo-humidified high-flow therapy promotes mucociliary clearance, secretion management, decreases dead space and provides stable FiO_2.

Several clinical trials have demonstrated its usefulness in the management of acute patients with hypoxemic respiratory failure, however, its use in other clinical conditions such as respiratory rehabilitation is still controversial. This chapter summarizes the use of thermo-humidified high-flow oxygen therapy in the COPD patient during physical activity.

Keywords: COPD, high-flow nasal cannula, oxygen therapy, high-intensity exercise, constant physical work, fraction of inspired oxygen (FiO_2), partial oxygen saturation (SpO_2)

Introduction

Chronic obstructive pulmonary disease (COPD) is one of the main causes of morbidity and mortality worldwide, the prevalence of which varies between

* Corresponding Author's Email: jonathan.camara@sjd.es.

In: Nasal High Flow and Non-Invasive Ventilatory Support
Editors: A. M. Esquinas, D. A. Lagonidis, P. Silva Santos et al.
ISBN: 979-8-88697-420-1

countries. The prevalence and global burden are expected to increase in the coming decades due to continued exposure to risk factors (smoking, environmental pollution) and aging population. COPD can lead to chronic respiratory failure, with concomitant hypoxia and hypercapnia, each of which is associated with a worse prognosis.

Respiratory rehabilitation, as defined by the American Thoracic Society/European Respiratory Society (ATS/ERS), is a comprehensive intervention based on patient assessment followed by tailored therapies including, but not limited to, exercise training, education, and body modifications designed to improve the physical and psychological condition of people with chronic respiratory diseases [1], which has well-established benefits in relation to exercise capacity, health-related quality of life and psychological well-being in patients with COPD.

Humidified high-flow nasal cannula (HFNC) is a type of non-invasive respiratory support that delivers gas through special nasal cannula, at flows greater than 30 L/min (up to 60 L/min), with controlled FiO_2 and under optimal conditions of temperature (31-37°C) and humidity (100% relative humidity, 44 mg H_2O/L absolute humidity) [2]. Numerous studies have investigated the physiological mechanisms that may explain some of the possible benefits of this modality compared to standard oxygen therapy, including Reduction of anatomical dead space, generation of positive end-expiratory pressure (PEEP), decreased work of breathing, constant FiO_2 delivery and improved mucociliary clearance [3].

The physiological effects of HFNC, combined with its simplicity and convenience, make the therapy an ideal candidate not only for long-term use, but also for respiratory support during COPD exacerbations and physical training during pulmonary rehabilitation. However, there are few data that support the widespread use of this therapy in respiratory rehabilitation units. This review aims to provide current evidence on the use of HFNC during respiratory rehabilitation in COPD patients based on available data.

Mechanisms by Which HFNC May Offer Advantages in Stable COPD

Improved Pulmonary Mucociliary Clearance

The air reaching main bronchi is moist [100% relative humidity (RH), absolute humidity (AH) = 44 mg/L] and warm (37°C). These humidity levels are reached due to the passage of air from the nasopharynx to a little below the carina (Isothermal Saturation Limit - ISB). Animal studies have shown that these conditions are optimal for maintaining normal epithelial cell function and that a reduction in air temperature alters their function [4]. As it is logical to think, at flows above the physiological ones, the upper airway is unable to heat and humidity the air, which leads to a deterioration of the ciliary function, with the consequent development of microatelectasis– atelectasis. The HFNC effectively delivers heated, humidified gas to the airways.

Anatomical Dead Space and CO_2 Washout

High-flow therapy allows greater removal of carbon dioxide (CO_2) and decreases dead space (Vd) attributable to exhaled volume, allowing a greater fraction of the tidal volume to be involved in hematosis. Moller and colleagues [5] have shown in two different upper airway models that high-flow therapy is able to decrease dead space by creating a reserve of air (oxygenated and lower CO_2) in the upper airway. Exercise intolerance in COPD is due in part to an elevated dead space, leading to a compensatory increase in minute ventilation [6].

PEEP Effect

High flow systems generate a non-constant level of positive pressure in the nasopharynx, depending on the flow used and the patient's breathing pattern (breath with mouth closed or open). This pressure ranges between 2-3 cm H_2O on average with flows between 35-60 L/min with open mouth and between 5-7 cm H_2O with closed mouth [7]. Inspiratory pressure and auto-PEEP counterbalancing, through the PEEP effect, could suggest a role in reducing the work of breathing, especially in COPD patients. This was demonstrated by Pisani et al., who compared the work in patients with alveolar hypoventilation secondary to COPD in stable phase treated with HFNC and standard oxygen therapy, showing a reduction in the transdiaphragmatic pressure oscillation (Pdi), in the pressure-time product of the diaphragm (PTPdi), as well as respiratory rate (RR) and $PaCO_2$ levels in those patients who were given high-flow therapy [8].

Decreased Inspiratory Resistance

It is known that in normal subjects [9], the inhalation of cold air causes the activation of specific receptors or osmoreceptors in the nasal mucosa, which induces bronchoconstriction. In COPD patients, inhalation of cold, dry air through the nasal mucosa can trigger bronchospasm through a mechanism mediated by the activation of muscarinic receptors [10]. Physiologically, the nasopharynx behaves as a conditioning of the inspired gas to be delivered to the alveolus in optimal conditions of heat and humidity, but also offers an anatomical resistance to its flow. High flow therapy tends to minimize this inspiratory resistance by administering flows that exceed the patient's peak inspiratory flow [11].

Airflow with Stable FiO_2

If the patient's ventilatory demand exceeds the flows provided by the device (nasal prongs, Venturi mask), the delivered FiO_2 would be unstable and lower than expected, due to the gaseous mixture with atmospheric air. For this reason, the actual FiO_2 is not stable during oxygen delivery with conventional methods. With HFNC, especially at high flow and closed-mouth breathing, the delivered flow is much higher than the patient's spontaneous inspiratory flow, so the actual FiO_2 is close to the predicted FiO_2 [12].

Use of the HFNC during Exercise

The review of the current literature allows us to collect different publications. Then, five full text articles were relevant and will be discussed separately. It is noteworthy that in all published studies, high-flow nasal cannula therapy was used during the physical activity sessions outlined in the research protocols. Now, there are no published studies where high flow therapy is an integral part of respiratory rehabilitation programs.

High-Flow Humidified Nasal Cannula (HFNC) Compared to Conventional Oxygen Therapy during a Single Constant Work Trial

Chalila et al., assessed exercise endurance with HFNC compared to conventional low-flow oxygen therapy in patients with COPD [13]. For this, 10 patients with severe COPD, without cardiovascular comorbidity, in a stable phase and without exacerbations in the last 3 months (average FEV_1 of 23 ± 6%, with chronic home oxygen therapy, average flow of 2 ± 1.6 lpm). These patients first underwent a constant work test without load, with O_2 by nasal cannula (average flow of 4 ± 1.8 bpm) for 12 minutes, followed by a 30-minute rest period. Subsequently, this test was repeated using HFNC with oral piece at a flow of 20 lpm and titratable FiO_2, in order to obtain a similar value to that used with conventional therapy. Each patient had an esophageal balloon catheter connected to a respiratory mechanics monitor along with a differential pressure/flow pneumotachograph. The following variables were measured: respiratory rate, tidal volume, minute volume, work of breathing, Ti/Ttot ratio, PTP (pressure-time product) and esophageal pressure swing, as well as dyspnea (assessed by the BORG scale), SpO_2, heart rate, blood pressure. The following results were obtained:

1. High flow vs low flow at rest: Better SpO_2 and PaO_2 values were obtained in the high flow group (98 ± 2 and 128 ± 34 mmHg respectively).
2. High flow vs. low flow during exercise: Only 5 patients completed the 12-minute session, due to dyspnea and fatigue. Of these, those who used high flow had better SpO_2 and PaO_2 values, lower respiratory rate and tolerated the sensation of dyspnea better. There were no differences in the values of tidal volume, minute volume, work of breathing, PTP.

The limitations of this study are clear, where the flow of 20 lpm used in the high-flow group stands out (considering that the concept in adults implies the use of flows above 30 lpm), the impossibility of accurately calculating FiO_2, the small sample and the fact that only five patients have completed the test.

High-Flow Humidified Nasal Cannula (HFNC) Compared to Conventional Oxygen Therapy during High-Intensity Constant Work Trial

Prieur et al., assessed 19 patients with severe/very severe COPD (FEV_1 28 ± 10%) recently discharged (less than 7 days) for COPD exacerbation, who underwent a high-intensity endurance test (80% of their maximum capacity) for 2 consecutive days, with low-flow oxygen therapy and high flow respectively (flow of 60 lpm, at 31°C and FiO_2 titratable to obtain SpO_2 above 90%) [14]. The primary objective was to measure endurance (duration of the test) in both conditions. As secondary objectives, SO_2 of the vastus lateralis muscle, degree of dyspnea, limb discomfort, transcutaneous pressure of CO_2 ($PtCO_2$), SpO_2, maximum inspiratory pressure (Pimax) and patient satisfaction were measured.

There was no difference in exercise tolerance between both groups and only three patients preferred high-flow therapy. The authors concluded that high-flow nasal cannula does not improve exercise tolerance in patients recovering from exacerbation.

High-Flow Humidified Nasal Cannula (HFNC) Compared to Venturi Mask Oxygen Therapy during a Single Constant Work Trial

To assess the effect of high-flow therapy in patients with severe COPD in stable phase (FEV_1 35 ± 12%, PaO_2 73 ± 13 mmHg, PCO_2 42 ± 5 mmHg), 2 constant work tests were performed at 75% of maximum load on 2 separate days: One day with HFNC and another with Venturi mask. FiO_2 remained constant during both trials, with values titrated to keep SpO_2 above 88%. The flow used was between 50 and 60 lpm in the high flow group [15]. The results showed greater resistance to exercise (in the duration of the test) in those patients who used the HFNC, with less sensation of dyspnea and limb fatigue. This improvement is partly explained by the decrease in dead space and the better supply of oxygen in relation to the patient's peak inspiratory flow. However, it´s noteworthy that the minute volume was not measured and that the FiO_2 in those patients who used the Venturi mask may be lower than expected.

High-Flow Humidified Nasal Cannula (HFNC) Compared to Venturi Mask Oxygen Therapy during a Single Constant Work Test and a Steady-Increment Work Trial

Dell'Era et al., evaluated 28 patients with COPD (FEV_1 44 ± 19%) with indication of oxygen therapy during physical exercise [16]. In these patients, both the maximum speed reached in the cycle ergometer as well as the resistance (duration of the test) were measured on two alternate days: 1 day with HFNC and another with oxygen therapy by Venturi mask, with recovery time between tests from 48 to 72 hours. The FiO_2 used was 40%.

Both variables (maximum speed and resistance) were greater in the group with high flow (5.9 vs. 5.7 Km/h and 450 vs. 315 seconds). With these data, the authors conclude that high-flow therapy is superior to Venturi mask oxygen therapy during a constant and progressively increasing physical effort test.

High Flow Humidified Nasal Cannula (HFNC) during Physical Exercise in Patients with COPD and Chronic Hypoxemia

Unlike previous studies, in this randomized clinical trial conducted by Vitacca et al., measurements were taken into account over 20 sessions with a cycle ergometer, spread over five per week. They included 171 patients with COPD and hypoxemic respiratory failure (carrying chronic home oxygen), in a stable phase of the disease and with no history of recent exacerbation [17]. All patients underwent a first test on the cycle ergometer with 50% of the maximum predicted load and breathing through a Venturi mask, with adjustable FiO_2 to maintain a target SpO_2 above 93%. Subsequently, two groups were randomized: one with Venturi mask oxygen therapy, and the other with high-flow nasal cannula.

No significant difference was obtained in the maximum tolerated load, heart rate, degree of dyspnea, tolerance to physical activity and SpO_2, but there was an increase in the distance covered in the 6-minute walk test in the group that used HFNC. Although no significant statistical difference was obtained between the two groups, the authors conclude that it is important to assess the clinical benefit that could be obtained, given the findings of the 6-minute walk test.

Conclusion

Of the studies presented, most show promising results in favor of the use of high-flow therapy during physical activity in patients with COPD, except for one in which the effect of recent exacerbation may lead to a lower response to therapy, due to the complexity of changes in the pathophysiology of the disease and how difficult it could be to titrate an adequate FiO_2.

However, the evidence supporting the widespread clinical use of AFHCN therapy during physical activity is still limited. A higher degree of evidence will be needed to incorporate this therapy into routine clinical practice, especially in a respiratory rehabilitation program.

References

[1] Andrews, S. M., M. Carter, H. Deoghare, P. K. Mills, K. Van Gundy, and V. V. Jain, "Pulmonary rehabilitation maintenance program prevents accelerated FEV1 decline and may prevent exacerbations in patients with severe COPD," *American Journal of Respiratory and Critical Care Medicine*, vol. 191, article A2013, 2015.

[2] Nishimura, M. High-flow nasal cannula oxygen therapy devices. *Breathe Care* 2019, 64, 735–742.

[3] Pisani, L., Vega, ML Use of nasal high flow in stable COPD: Rationale and physiology. *COPD J. Chronic Obstr Pulm. Dis.* 2017, 14, 1–5.

[4] Kilgour, E., Rankin N., Ryan S., Pack R. Mucociliary function deteriorates in the clinical range of inspired air temperature and humidity. *Intense Care Med* 2004; 30:1491–1494.

[5] Möller, W., Celik G., Feng S., Bartenstein P., Meyer G., Oliver E., Otmar Schmid, Stanislav Tatkov. Nasal high flow clears anatomical dead space in upper airway models. *J Appl Physiol* (1985) 2015; 118:1525–532.

[6] Elbehairy, A. F., Ciavaglia C. E., Webb K. A., Guenette J. A., Jensen D., Mourad S. M., J. Alberto Neder, and Denis E. O'Donnel. Pulmonary gas exchange abnormalities in mild chronic obstructive pulmonary disease. Implications for dyspnea and exercise intolerance. *Am J Respir Crit Care Med.* 2015 June; 191:1384–1394.

[7] Parke, R., McGuinness S., Eccleston M. Nasal high-flow therapy delivers low level positive airway pressure. *Br J Anaesth* 2009; 103:886–890.

[8] Pisani, L., Fasano L., Corcione N., Comellini V., Musti M. A., Brandao M., Bottone D., Calderini E., Navalesi P., Nava S. Change in pulmonary mechanics and the effect on breathing pattern of high flow oxygen therapy in stable hypercapnic COPD. *Thorax* 2017; 72:373–375.

[9] Fontanari, P., Burnet H., Zattara-Hartmann M. C., Jammes Y. Changes in airway resistance induced by nasal inhalation of cold dry, dry, or moist air in normal individuals. *J Appl Physiol* 1996; 81(4):1739–1743.

[10] On, L. S., Boonyongsunchai P., Webb S., Davies L., Calverley P. M., Costello R. W. Function of pulmonary neuronal M(2) muscarinic receptors in stable chronic obstructive pulmonary disease. *Am J Respir Crit Care Med* 2001; 163(6):1320–1325.

[11] Fraser, J. F., Spooner A. J., Dunster K. R., Anstey C. M., Corley A. Nasal high flow oxygen therapy in patients with COPD reduces respiratory rate and tissue carbon dioxide while increasing tidal and end-expiratory lung volumes: a randomized crossover trial. *Thorax* 2016; 71:759–761.

[12] Ritchie, J. E., Williams A. B., Gerard C., Hockey H. Evaluation of a humidified nasal high-flow oxygen system, using oxygraphy, capnography and measurement of upper airway pressures. *Anaesth Intensive Care* 2011; 39:1103–1110.

[13] Chatila, W., Nugent T., Vance G., Gaughan J., Criner G. J. The effects of high-flow vs. low-flow oxygen on exercise in advanced obstructive airways disease. *Chest.* 2004 Oct; 126(4):1108–15.

[14] Prieur, G., Medrinal C., Combret Y., Dupuis Lozeron E., Bonnevie T., Gravier F. E., Quieffin, Bouchra J. E., Lamia, Jean-Christian Borel, Reychler G. Nasal high flow does not improve exercise tolerance in COPD patients recovering from acute exacerbation: A randomized crossover study. *Respirology.* 2019 Nov; 24(11): 1088–94.

[15] Cirio, S., Piran M., Vitacca M., Piaggi G., Ceriana P., Prazzoli M., Paneroni M., Carlucci A. Effects of heated and humidified high flow gases during high-intensity constant-load exercise on severe COPD patients with ventilatory limitation. *Respir Med.* 2016 Sep; 118: 128–32.

[16] Dell'Era, S., Nicolas R., Elena G. S., Sergio T. The High Flow Nasal Cannula Improves the Exercise Capacity in Patients with Chronic Obstructive Pulmonary Disease: Randomized, Crossover Clinical Trial. *Rev Am Med Respir.* 2019; 19(1): 16–26.

[17] Vitacca, M., Paneroni M., Zampogna, Visca D. High-Flow Oxygen Therapy During Exercise Training in Patients With Chronic Obstructive Pulmonary Disease and Chronic Hypoxemia: A Multicenter Randomized Controlled Trial. *Phys Ther.* 2020;12;100(8):1249-1259.

Chapter 9

Adverse Effects in High-Flow Nasal Cannula Oxygen Therapy

Sara Morgado*, MD

Pulmonology Unit, West Lisbon Hospital Center,
Egas Moniz Hospitals, Lisboa, Portugal

Abstract

Oxygen therapy is the primary treatment for hypoxemic respiratory failure. Oxygen is typically delivered through conventional low- or high-flow systems, which do not provide a consistent fraction of inspired oxygen. Thus, to overcome this problem, the high-flow nasal cannula oxygen therapy was created, which consists of a non-invasive respiratory support therapy that provides to the patient heated, and humidified air enriched with oxygen in a reliable fraction. This chapter addresses the main adverse effects related to this therapy, namely according to age group, and its most important limitations, as per the literature.

Keywords: respiratory failure, respiratory therapy, high-flow nasal cannula oxygen therapy, adverse effects, limitations

Introduction

Acute respiratory failure is one of the main causes of mortality, especially in Intensive Care Units, with oxygen therapy being the first-line treatment [1]. In conventional oxygen therapy devices, which include nasal cannulas, simple

* Corresponding Author's Email: saragmorgado@gmail.com.

In: Nasal High Flow and Non-Invasive Ventilatory Support
Editors: A. M. Esquinas, D. A. Lagonidis, P. Silva Santos et al.
ISBN: 979-8-88697-420-1

face masks, Venturi masks and masks with a high concentration reservoir, the maximum flow rate that can be achieved is only 15 L/min, which is lower than the inspiratory flow of mostly of the patients with acute respiratory failure [1]. In addition, these devices present other disadvantages, such as limiting the fraction of inspired oxygen (FiO_2) and insufficient humidification and heating of the inspired gas, causing discomfort to the patient [2]. High-flow nasal cannula (HFNC) oxygen therapy delivers heated and humidified oxygen via the nasal or tracheal route, reaching flow rates up to 60 L/min [1, 2, 3, 4].

HFNC was initially widely used in neonates and children, but lately, it has been increasingly used in adults, with clinical benefit [4]. The advantages of HFNC compared to conventional oxygen therapies include greater comfort, greater humidification of secretions to facilitate their elimination, decreased anatomical dead space to improve ventilation efficiency, providing a small positive pressure effect on the airways, and high flow rates, to minimize mixing with outdoor air for more accurate FiO_2 [3, 5]. Furthermore, it is easy to use and apply [2, 3, 5].

HFNC can then be an alternative to conventional oxygen therapy and non-invasive ventilation (NIV) [4], namely, in hypoxemic respiratory failure, in hypercapnic respiratory failure [6], after extubation, before and during intubation, in postoperative respiratory failure, during bronchoscopy, in acute heart failure, among others [1, 2, 3, 5].

HFNC has been used successfully in several clinical situations, however, there are no defined recommendations for its application in clinical practice. Therefore, its proven benefit is subjective, based on physiological outcomes, which are not always reflected in improved clinical results neither in heterogeneous population trial studies [1, 2, 3, 5].

Adverse Effects

When HFNC is applied at a very high flow, humidification may be inadequate, thus causing dryness of the nasal mucosa, mouth, and throat, eye irritation, and epistaxis [3, 7, 8].

Age Groups

Premature Newborns

In the case of premature babies, the main adverse effects of HFNC were nasal mucosa damage and pneumothorax [7]. However, in a randomized controlled trial including preterm infants younger than 32 weeks, nasal trauma was less frequent in the HFNC group compared to the Continuous Positive Airway Pressure group (CPAP) [9].

Children

In the case of children, in most of the studies, they tolerated well the treatment, with few adverse effects being reported. Therefore, concluding that its use is safe in this age group [9, 10]. However, two studies described four cases of pneumothorax in children under HFNC: a 2-month-old child with respiratory syncytial virus bronchiolitis under HFNC with a flow rate of 6–8 L/min; a 16-year-old child with cerebral palsy under HFNC with a flow rate of 15–20 L/min; a 22-month-old boy with a subdural hematoma under HFNC with a flow rate of 6 L/min); a 4-year-old child with asthma treated with HFNC with a flow of 40 L/min [3, 9]. Furthermore, HFNC should be used with caution in children with intra-abdominal pathology, as three studies reported abdominal distention in children with HFNC [9]. Other adverse effects reported were nasal mucosa damage with epistaxis and ulceration [9].

Adults

Most adults tolerate HFNC, and its adverse effects are rare in this age group [5, 11]. Regarding the use of HFNC in an outpatient setting, namely in patients with Chronic Obstructive Pulmonary Disease (COPD), a study revealed that during 12 months of treatment no adverse events were recorded [12]. Concerning its use for respiratory support in adults in Intensive Care Units, in a Cochrane systematic review, some of the possible adverse effects of HFNC were analyzed.

Compared to conventional oxygen therapy, in terms of pneumonia cases, HFNC results in slight or no difference (RR 0.72, 95% CI 0.48 to 1.09; 4 studies, 1057 participants; evidence of moderate certainty). Regarding nasal mucosa injury or skin trauma, it is not possible to be sure of the effect of HFNC because the certainty of the evidence for this result is very low (RR 3.66, 95% CI 0.43 to 31.48; 2 studies, 617 participants; very low certainty evidence) [9]. Compared to non-invasive mechanical ventilation, for pneumonia cases, it is not possible to be sure about the effect of the use of HFNC on its incidence, due to very low certainty evidence (RR 0.51, 95% CI 0.17 to 1.52; 3 studies, 1,750 participants; very low certainty evidence); in terms of nasal mucosa injury or skin trauma, none of the studies analyzed reported data for this outcome. Regarding barotrauma, there has not been found any evidence of difference in the incidence of pneumothorax under HFNC (RR 1.15, 95% CI 0.42 to 3.14; 1 study, 830 participants; low certainty evidence) [13].

Limitations

Open System

According to some studies, the HFNC is an open system, that is, it does not push or extract respiratory gases from the lungs, and, consequently, it does not improve tidal volume or ventilation per minute, verifying that the tidal volume was constant. and respiratory rate was reduced, with lower minute ventilation [2, 3].

Inaccurate FiO_2 with Mouth Opening

In the HFNC, the high flow rates result in minimal outdoor air intake, resulting in a more accurate delivery of oxygen, especially when compared to conventional oxygen therapy systems. However, breathing with an open mouth or breathing during exercise somehow slightly mitigate this advantage [2, 5].

Loss of Positive Airway Pressure Effect with Mouth Opening

Several studies have shown that, although the HFNC is an open system, the high flow of the nasal cannula increases the nasopharyngeal airway pressure that peaks at the end of expiration, decreasing the work of breathing and improving oxygenation [5]. According to Richie et al., the HFNC can provide clinically relevant positive airway pressure, directly proportional to the oxygen flow rates provided. Also depending on the size of the nasal cannula in relation to the nostrils, and high flows can function as a resistance to expiration when the mouth is closed boosting the HFNC effect. According to

Parke et al., for each 10 L/minute increase in HFNC flow rate, mean airway pressure increased by 0.69 cmH_2O ($p < 0.01$) when individuals breathed with mouth closed and 0.35 cmH_2O ($p < 0.03$) with mouth open [2, 5, 8].

Humidification Loss at Very High-Flow Rates

When HFNC is applied at very high flow, humidification may be less adequate. Although these devices incorporate a heated humidifier into the mechanical ventilation system, the ability of such systems to create adequate vapor at a high flow rate remains unclear [3].

Absence of Pressure Relief Valves for Adults

Pediatric HFNC systems incorporate safety valves to prevent high pressures. Nevertheless, adult systems do not have a pressure relief valve or pressure monitors, and it is not possible to regulate or determine the pressure applied into the airways which can lead to barotrauma in the case of very high pressures [3, 9].

Masks Clinical Worsening

Recognition of acute respiratory distress syndrome (ARDS) may be hampered by HFNC because the improvements in oxygenation seen in mild ARDS may result in an arterial blood oxygen partial pressure (PaO2)/FiO_2 ratio below the diagnostic threshold, without considering the positive end-expiratory effect of HFNC. Thus, it could potentially delay necessary intubation and worsen some results such as mortality [5]. Furthermore, as HFNC is more comfortable for patients than NIV, it can be tolerated for longer periods of time, which may neglect the need for intubation [2].

High Cost

The HFNC has a high cost in terms of energy, due to the humidification and heating process. As an example, under normal conditions (ambient temperature of 21°C with 50% relative humidity), an adult person breathing with a tidal volume of 500 mL and a respiratory rate of 12 breaths/minute may require about 156 calories/minute for conditioning the inspired gas. Thus, in the case of a patient with a pulmonary disorder, due to the increase in ventilation/minute, the amount of air to be humidified and heated is even greater, conveying to higher costs [8].

Conclusion

HFNC corresponds to a non-invasive respiratory support therapy that guarantees adequate oxygenation and alveolar ventilation. This therapy is well tolerated by neonates, children, and adults with hypoxemic respiratory failure. In general, its adverse effects are rare and appear in smaller numbers compared to other therapies. There is a lack of information in the literature regarding the adverse effects of HFNC, given that it is a recent therapy. Therefore, further studies in this area are important, as well as for the definition of concrete indications for HFNC and objective criteria for initiation, and discontinuation of this type of therapy.

In summary, HNFC is increasingly used as respiratory support therapy, and HNFC is well tolerated by most of the patients. The main adverse effects described were dryness of the nasal mucosa, mouth and throat, eye irritation, epistaxis, nasal mucosa injury, facial skin trauma, pneumothorax, abdominal distension, and pneumonia. The HNFC also has some limitations, most of which are related to mouth opening or the high flow rates applied. More studies focusing on the potential adverse effects of this therapy are needed, hence the current scientific evidence is limited.

References

[1] Xu, Z., Li, Y., Zhou, J., Li, X., Huang, Y., Liu, X., Zhang, H. 2018. "High-flow nasal cannula in adults with acute respiratory failure and after extubation: a systematic review and meta-analysis." *Respiratory Research*, 19(1). doi:10.1186/s12931-018-0907.

[2] Papazian, L., Corley, A., Hess, D., Fraser, J. F., Frat, J. P., Guitton, C., Azoulay, E. 2016. "Use of high-flow nasal cannula oxygenation in ICU adults: a narrative review." *Intensive Care Medicine*, 42(9), 1336–1349. doi:10.1007/s00134-016-4277-8.

[3] Nishimura, M. 2016. "High-Flow Nasal Cannula Oxygen Therapy in Adults: Physiological Benefits, Indication, Clinical Benefits, and Adverse Effects." *Respiratory Care*, 61(4), 529–541. doi:10.4187/respcare.04577.

[4] Huang, H.-W., Sun, X.-M., Shi, Z.-H., Chen, G.-Q., Chen, L., Friedrich, J. O., and Zhou, J.-X. 2017. "Effect of High-Flow Nasal Cannula Oxygen Therapy Versus Conventional Oxygen Therapy and Noninvasive Ventilation on Reintubation Rate in Adult Patients After Extubation: A Systematic Review and Meta-Analysis of Randomized Controlled Trials." *Journal of Intensive Care Medicine*, 08850666 1770511. doi:10.1177/0885066617705118.

[5] Hyzy, Robert. 2021. *Heated and humidified high-flow nasal oxygen in adults: Practical considerations and potential applications.* UpToDate. Accessed October 2021. https://www.uptodate.com/contents/heated-and-humidified-high-flow-nasal-oxygen-in-adults-practical-considerations-and-potential-applications#H86757176 0.

[6] Sun, J., Li, Y., Ling, B., Zhu, Q., Hu, Y., Tan, D., Xu, J. 2019. "High flow nasal cannula oxygen therapy versus non-invasive ventilation for chronic obstructive pulmonary disease with acute-moderate hypercapnic respiratory failure: an observational cohort study." *International Journal of Chronic Obstructive Pulmonary Disease*, Volume 14, 1229–1237. doi:10.2147/copd.s206567 .

[7] Farley, R. C., Hough, J. L., and Jardine, L. A. 2015. "Strategies for the discontinuation of humidified high flow nasal cannula (HHFNC) in preterm infants." *Cochrane Database of Systematic Reviews.* doi:10.1002/14651858. cd01 1079.pub2.

[8] Pisani, L., and Vega, M. L. 2017. "Use of Nasal High Flow in Stable COPD: Rationale and Physiology." *COPD: Journal of Chronic Obstructive Pulmonary Disease*, 14(3), 346–350. doi:10.1080/15412555.2017.1315.

[9] Mikalsen, I. B., Davis, P., and Øymar, K. 2016. "High flow nasal cannula in children: a literature review." *Scandinavian Journal of Trauma, Resuscitation and Emergency Medicine*, 24(1). doi:10.1186/s13049-016-0278-4 .

[10] Beggs, S., Wong, Z. H., Kaul, S., Ogden, K. J., and Walters, J. A. 2014. "High-flow nasal cannula therapy for infants with bronchiolitis." *Cochrane Database of Systematic Reviews.* doi:10.1002/14651858.cd009609.pub2 .

[11] Hernández, G., Vaquero, C., Colinas, L., Cuena, R., González, P., Canabal, A., Fernández, R. 2016. "Effect of Postextubation High-Flow Nasal Cannula vs Noninvasive Ventilation on Reintubation and Postextubation Respiratory Failure in High-Risk Patients." *JAMA*, 316(15), 1565. doi:10.1001/jama.2016.14194.

[12] Storgaard, L. H., Hockey, H., Laursen, B. S., and Weinreich, U. M. 2018. "Long-term effects of oxygen-enriched high-flow nasal cannula treatment in COPD patients with chronic hypoxemic respiratory failure." *International Journal of Chronic Obstructive Pulmonary Disease*, Volume 13, 1195–1205. doi:10.2147/ copd.s159666.

[13] Lewis, S. R., Baker, P. E., Parker, R., and Smith, A. F. 2021. "High-flow nasal cannulae for respiratory support in adult intensive care patients." *Cochrane Database of Systematic Reviews*, 021(3). doi:10.1002/14651858.cd010172.pub3.

Chapter 10

Contraindications for High-Flow Nasal Oxygen Therapy

Nuno Faria[1,2,*], MD
and Cláudia Sofia Alves[2], MD
[1] Pulmonology Service, Porto Hospital and University Center, Porto, Portugal
[2] Institute of Biomedical Sciences Abel Salazar, University of Porto, Porto, Portugal

Abstract

High-flow nasal cannula (HFNC) delivers heated (31-37ºC), humidified oxygen at high flows with a consistent percentage of inspired oxygen (FiO_2) of 0.21-1.00. The interface commonly employed is a nasal cannula, which provides comfort and less claustrophobic feeling than the face/nasal masks conventionally used in NIV. To date there is no scientific evidence to establish absolute contraindications for applying HFNC.

Regarding relative contraindications, it is important to highlight that HFNC should not delay advanced airway management in a patient requiring immediate endotracheal intubation. This applies to patients with an acutely impaired mental status, risk of aspiration, upper airway abnormalities or another situation that prompts the need for airway protection. Complications are rare but may include local trauma/ discomfort, abdominal distension, aspiration, epistaxis and barotrauma, though these occur less commonly than with NIV. As predictors of HFNC failure, low peripheral oxygen saturation, high respiratory rate and thoracoabdominal asynchrony should be considered.

The ROX index has been proposed as a useful tool to predict HFNC failure/success. Successful HFNC is expected when ROX index is above

* Corresponding Author's Email: nunofaria.pneumologia@chporto.min-saude.pt.

In: Nasal High Flow and Non-Invasive Ventilatory Support
Editors: A. M. Esquinas, D. A. Lagonidis, P. Silva Santos et al.
ISBN: 979-8-88697-420-1

4.88 (either at 2,6 or 12h) and HFNC failure is expected when ROX index is below 3.85 (ROX index between 3.85 and 4.88 should be reassessed in 1- 2h).

In summary, relative contraindications for HFNC include but are not limited to upper airway abnormalities, hemodynamic instability, life-threatening hypoxia, skull base trauma, and pneumothorax, which can lead to HFNC ineffectiveness or make it potentially dangerous.

Keywords: high-flow nasal cannula, contraindications, ROX index, NIV, COVID-19

Introduction

High flow nasal cannula (HFNC) delivers heated (31-37ºC), humidified (until 100% relative humidity) oxygen at high flows with a consistent percentage of inspired oxygen (FiO_2) of 0.21-1.00. This enhances oxygenation, lowers airway resistance, offers humidified flow to cleanse anatomical dead space and gives a modest level of positive end expiratory pressure (PEEP). The interface commonly employed is a nasal cannula, which provides comfort and less claustrophobic feeling than the face/nasal masks conventionally used in NIV [1]. HFNC oxygen therapy is therefore well tolerated by most patients.

To date there is no scientific evidence to establish absolute contraindications for applying HFNC [2]. Regarding relative contra-indications, it is important to highlight that HFNC should not delay advanced airway management in a patient requiring immediate endotracheal intubation. This applies to patients with an acutely impaired mental status, risk of aspiration, upper airway abnormalities or another situation that that prompts the need for airway protection [3, 4] (Table 1).

Many of the contraindications mentioned in Table 1 are related to the proper fitting of the nasal prongs, namely facial, nose or airway anomalies or other lesions that alter the structure of the facial mass [1, 5]. Therefore, it is crucial to evaluate any deformities in the face, nose, or airway, including epistaxis, basilar skull fracture, nose or upper aerodigestive tract surgery or any cause of significant nasal obstruction. Nevertheless, in patients with facial structure/hair resulting in air leakage or difficulty adapting to a facial interface, HFNC may be a viable alternative to non-invasive ventilation (NIV) [6, 7].

Table 1. Relative contraindications to high-flow nasal cannula in adults [3–5, 8, 9]

Upper airway obstruction
Nasal obstruction e.g., tumor, polyps, septal deformity/trauma
Blocked nasal airway e.g., choanal atresia
Foreign body aspiration
Copious, unmanageable respiratory secretions
Severe oropharyngeal mucositis
Trauma or surgery to nasopharynx
Trauma (maxillofacial/suspected base of skull fracture/chest)
Facial burns/trauma/recent facial or upper airway surgery*
Epistaxis
Central apnea
Life-threatening hypoxia
Life threatening apneas/hemodynamic instability
Life-threatening dysrhythmias
Pneumothorax
Inability to protect own airway
Decreased level of consciousness (LOC)

* Some experts avoid HFNC in those following upper airway surgery to avoid the theoretical risk that the high pressure may precipitate a venous thromboembolism [5].

Complications are rare but may include local trauma/discomfort, abdominal distension, aspiration, epistaxis, and barotrauma, though these occur less commonly than with NIV. The most significant and to avoid complication is delay in intubation and consequent worse clinical outcomes in patients with acute respiratory failure [1]. HFNC failure is less likely to increase mortality in the short term (i.e., < 24 h), therefore a trial in the emergency department is appropriate in selected patients with acute hypoxemic respiratory failure.

As predictors of HFNC failure, low peripheral oxygen saturation, high respiratory rate and thoracoabdominal asynchrony should be considered [6]. The ROX index has been proposed as a useful tool to predict HFNC failure/success. This index is calculated as the ratio of pulse oximetry oxygen saturation to the fraction of inspired oxygen [SpO_2/FiO_2)/RR]. Successful HFNC is expected when ROX index is above 4.88 (either at 2,6 or 12h) and HFNC failure is expected when ROX index is below 3.85 (ROX index between 3.85 and 4.88 should be reassessed in 1-2h) [1]. Although the exact time to stop HFNC and increase respiratory support is not standardized, this decision must be made by the patient's care team [3].

The relative contraindications for HFNC in children are similar to those in adults, with a special concern for the characteristic pathologies of this age group (Table 2). HFNC should be applied carefully in children with congenital heart disease or chronic respiratory failure. A well-known complication of HFNC in children is barotrauma such as air-trapping, pneumothorax, and pneumomediastinum. This occurs more frequently when an improperly large cannula is used. Nevertheless, serious pneumothorax in children is infrequent, although it has been reported even in low-flow settings [10].

Table 2. Relative contraindications to high flow nasal cannula in children [4, 6, 9, 11–14]. Same applied to adults (see Table 1)

Active vomiting Bowel obstruction Existing air leak e.g., pneumothorax or pneumomediastinum
Agitation or confusion predicting inability to tolerate
Infants with non-repaired gastro-intestinal obstructions e.g., tracheoesophageal fistula (TOF), Duodenal Atresia or Volvulus Congenital heart disease Certain craniofacial malformations Infants or children with non-patent nasal passages Infants weighing < 3 kg

* Some patients with congenital heart disease may be suitable candidates for HFNC therapy [14]. However, before starting therapy with HFNC it is necessary to discuss the case with the pediatric cardiologist in advance and carry out further investigations/necessary treatments [14]. The possibility of informing the pediatric intensive care unit (PICU) should also be considered [14].

COVID-19 is not a contraindication to HFNC [14]. Nevertheless, if SARS-CoV-2 infection is suspected or confirmed in a patient with respiratory distress and it is considered that the HFNC is necessary to optimize its management, complete personal protective equipment must be worn, and all local control policies must be adhered to [14]. ROX index below 4.88 at 2h seems also to predict HFNC failure in COVID-19 patients [1].

Conclusion

Relative contraindications for HFNC include but are not limited to upper airway abnormalities, hemodynamic instability, life-threatening hypoxia, skull base trauma, and pneumothorax, which can lead to HFNC ineffectiveness or make it potentially dangerous [10]. Since lower positive pressures are generally applied through HFNC than NIV, a lower frequency of side effects such as abdominal distension and barotrauma is expected [6]. When claustrophobic sensations or intolerance of tight interface contact are the main contraindications for NIV, HFNC is often a viable alternative [2, 15].

References

[1] Long B., S. Y. Liang, and S. Lentz, "High flow nasal cannula for adult acute hypoxemic respiratory failure in the ED setting," *The American Journal of Emergency Medicine*, vol. 49, pp. 352–359, Nov. 2021, doi: 10.1016/j.ajem.2021.06.074.

[2] Nishimura M., "High-flow nasal cannula oxygen therapy in adults," *J. Intensive Care*, vol. 3, no. 1, p. 15, Dec. 2015, doi: 10.1186/s40560-015-0084-5.

[3] Nagler Joshua, MD, MHPEd, "High-flow nasal cannula oxygen therapy in children," *UpToDate*. https://www.uptodate.com/contents/high-flow-nasal-cannula-oxygen-therapy-in-children?search=hight%20flow%20nasal%20cannula&source=search_result&selectedTitle=2~69&usage_type=default&display_rank=2 (accessed Nov. 28, 2021).

[4] Carlucci A. and S. M. Maggiore, Eds., *High Flow Nasal Cannula: Physiological Effects and Clinical Applications*. Cham: Springer International Publishing, 2021. doi: 10.1007/978-3-030-42454-1.

[5] Hyzy R. C., MD, "Heated and humidified high-flow nasal oxygen in adults: Practical considerations and potential applications," *UpToDate*. https://www.uptodate.com/contents/heated-and-humidified-high-flow-nasal-oxygen-in-adults-practical-considerations-and-potential-applications?search=hight%20flow%20nasal%20cannula&source=search_result&selectedTitle=1~69&usage_type=default&display_rank=1 (accessed Nov. 28, 2021).

[6] Spicuzza L. and M. Schisano, "High-flow nasal cannula oxygen therapy as an emerging option for respiratory failure: the present and the future," *Therapeutic Advances in Chronic Disease*, vol. 11, p. 204062232092010, Jan. 2020, doi: 10.1177/2040622320920106.

[7] Oczkowski S., Ergan B., Bos L., Chatwin M., Ferrer M., Gregoretti C., Heunks L., Frat J. P., Longhini F., Nava S., Navalesi P., Ozsancak Uğurlu A., Pisani L., Renda T., Thille A. W., Winck J. C., Windisch W., Tonia T., Boyd J., Sotgiu G., Scala R., "ERS Clinical Practice Guidelines: high-flow nasal cannula in acute respiratory failure," *European Respiratory Journal*, 2021, doi: 10.1183/13993003.01574-2021.

[8] *"High flow nasal prong (HFNP) therapy."* Accessed: Nov. 28, 2021. [Online]. Available: https://www.rch.org.au/rchcpg/hospital_clinical_guideline_index/High_flow_nasal_prong_(HFNP)_therapy/#contraindications.

[9] Perth Children's Hospital. *Humidified High Flow Nasal Cannula Therapy*. Accessed: Nov. 28, 2021. [Online]. Available: https://pch.health.wa.gov.au/For-

health-professionals/Clinical-Practice-Guidelines/Humidified-High-Flow-Nasal-Cannula-Therapy.

[10] Kwon J.-W., "High-flow nasal cannula oxygen therapy in children: a clinical review," *Clin. Exp. Pediatr.*, vol. 63, no. 1, pp. 3–7, Jan. 2020, doi: 10.3345/kjp.2019.00626.

[11] Hoffman E., K. L. Reichmuth, and M. L. Cooke, "A review of the use of high-flow nasal cannula oxygen therapy in hospitalised children at a regional hospital in the Cape Town Metro, South Africa," *S. Afr. Med. J.*, vol. 109, no. 4, p. 272, Mar. 2019, doi: 10.7196/SAMJ.2019.v109i4.13145.

[12] Tracey Couttie - Paediatric CNC, *Infants and children Humidified High-Flow Nasal Cannula Oxygen.* Mar. 2016. [Online]. https://www.medfromtheshed.com.au/uploads/6/7/6/2/67622653/islhd-clin-gl-17-infantsandchildrenhumidifiedhigh-flownasalcannulaoxygen.pdf.

[13] Agency for Clinical Innovation, *Humidified High Flow Nasal Cannula Oxygen Guideline for Metropolitan Paediatric Wards and EDs.* Jan. 29, 2016. [Online]. https://www1.health.nsw.gov.au/pds/ActivePDSDocuments/GL2016_004.pdf.

[14] [Online]. http://olchc-uat.ptools.net/healthcare-professionals/clinical-guidelines/humidified-high-flow-nasal-cannula-hhfnc-guideline.pdf.

[15] Nishimura M., "High-Flow Nasal Cannula Oxygen Therapy in Adults: Physiological Benefits, Indication, Clinical Benefits, and Adverse Effects," *Respiratory Care*, vol. 61, no. 4, pp. 529–541, Apr. 2016, doi: 10.4187/respcare.04577.

Chapter 11

Acute Hypoxemic Respiratory Failure: Pneumonia

Özlem Özkan Kuşcu[1,*]
and Ferit Kuşcu[2]
[1] Seyhan State Hospital, Intensive Care Unit, Adana, Turkey
[2] Cukurova University Medical Faculty,
Infecitous Diseases and Clinical Microbiology, Adana, Turkey

Abstract

Pneumonia is the infection of the pulmonary parenchyma. Patients with pneumonia may experience respiratory distress. In this case respiratory support with positive airway pressure is necessary. Positive airway pressure recruits collapsed alveoli and improves gas exchange with healing intrathoracic shunt and ventilation/perfusion rate, increases functional residual capacity and compliance. As a result work of breathing decreases with positive airway pressure. Respiratory support may be applied to the patients with non-invasive or invasive methods. In this chapter, non-invasive positive pressure use in pneumonia is detailed.

Keywords: pneumonia, respiratory distress, non-invasive mechanical ventilation, pneumonia/SDRA

[*] Corresponding Author's Email: ozlemozkankuscu@gmail.com.

In: Nasal High Flow and Non-Invasive Ventilatory Support
Editors: A. M. Esquinas, D. A. Lagonidis, P. Silva Santos et al.
ISBN: 979-8-88697-420-1

Introduction

Pneumonia is the infection of the pulmonary parenchyma and an important cause of morbidity and mortality [1, 2], can develop due to specific infectious or non-infectious etiologies, complications of diseases and procedures each with a different epidemiology, pathogenesis, presentation and clinical course [3]. Hippocrates first described pneumonia in BC 460-370 [4]. It's clinical and pathological features were descripted first by Laennec in 1819 [5]. Rokitansky was differentiated lobar and bronchopneumonia in 1842 [6].

Specific Diagnoses in Pneumonia

Pneumonia is classified, according to the anatomical placement, nonsegmental alveolar (lobar) pneumonia is also called non-segmental pneumonia or focal non-segmental pneumonia. There is a homogeneous and fibrinosuppurative consolidation in one or more lobes of a lung in response to bacterial pneumonia. *Streptococcus pneumoniae* is the most common causative organism of lobar pneumonia [7].

Bronchopneumonia (lobular pneumonia) is an acute inflammation of the bronchi with multiple consolidation foci in the pulmonary lobule or lobules [8]. Interstitial pneumonia: Idiopatic pulmonary fibrosis is the most common type. Normal lung, interstitial inflammation, fibrosis, and honeycomb replacement areas are the main diagnostic criteria [9].

Cryptogenic organizing pneumonia (COP) is noninfectious type of pneumonia with unknown etiology. Inflammation of bronchioles and the surrounding structures are the main diagnostic criteria [10].

According to the Etiology

Infectious

Pneumonia Bacterial

Streptococcus pneumoniae is the most common cause of bacterial pneumonia. *Mycoplasma pneumoniae*, *Haemophilus influenzae* and *Legionella pneumophila* are the other less common causes [11].

Viral

Respiratory viruses are the common cause of pneumonia. Influenza virus A and B, respiratory synctial virus, rhinoviruses, severe acute respiratory syndrome coronavirus 2 (SARS-CoV-2) are the other causative pathogens [12].

Fungal Pneumonia

Fungal pneumonia is the infection of the lungs, can be caused by either endemic or opportunistic fungi or a combination of both. In immunocompromised patients mortality of fungal pneumonias can be as high as 90%. *Pneumocystis jirovecii*, *Cryptococcus* species, Histoplasmosis species are the examples of fungi that can cause pneumonia [13].

Non-Infectious

Chemical Pneumonia

Is rare, may be acute or chronic, non-infectious, can be caused by inhalation or aspiration of irritants [14].

According to the Clinical Picture

Typical pneumonia is distinguished from atypical pneumonia by sudden onset of symptoms and lobar infiltration. Severe weakness, high fever and chills, purulent productive cough, tachypnea and shortness of breath, pleuritic chest pain that often accompanies pleural effusion while breathing are the common symptoms [15]. Atypical pneumonia is known as walking pneumonia because of mild symptoms. Intracelluler living bacteria are the common causative pathogens [16].

According to the Empirical Treatment Approach

Community acquired pneumonia is the most common type of pneumonia that occurs outside of the health care facilities. It may be caused by bacteria, bacteria like organisms, fungal and viral infections [17].

Hospital-acquired pneumonia (Healthcare-associated pneumonia, Ventilator-related pneumonia). Pneumonia developing at least 48-72 hours after hospitalization is defined as hospital acquired pneumonia or nosocomial pneumonia. Bacterial infection is the common cause [18].

Pneumonia Developed in Immunocompromised Patients

Immunocompromised patients are vulnerable to infections. Immunodeficiency may be congenital or may develop due to acquired immunodeficiency. Although survival has improved, pneumonia is the most common invasive infection with a high mortality and morbidity rate for immunocompromised patients [19]. According to the severity: Where a patient diagnosed with pneumonia should be treated is one of the most important factor for managing the disease process. This is necessary for patient outcomes and cost. Therefore scoring systems such as PSI, CURB-65 have been developed to determine the pneumonia severity [20].

Others

Aspiration pneumonia can develop as a part of community and hospital acquired pneumonia [21]. It is estimated that 5 to 15% of community-acquired pneumonia cases accounts for aspiration pneumonia. Microaspiration of a small amount of oropharyngeal secretion may occur during sleep in the healthy population [22]. However, this situation is the main pathogenetic mechanism in the development of pneumonia [23].

Pneumonia Developing in the Elderly

Pneumonia is common and severe problem in the elderly. Disease severity is strongly associated with age and age-related comorbidities. While Streptococcus pneumoniae is the main pathogen responsible for pneumonia in the elderly, anaerobic pathogens should be considered as causative [24].

Respiratory support should be required in patients who cannot be adequately respond to etiology-oriented pneumonia treatment. In this case, respiratory support can be applied with non-invasive and invasive methods. The physiological effects of positive pressure mechanical ventilation should also be taken into account in patients who will undergo respiratory support.

Effects of Positive Airway Pressure on the Circulatory System

Effects of Continuous Positive Airway Pressure (CPAP) on the cardiovascular system in patients with pneumonia are less known. Positive End Expiratuar Pressure (PEEP) increases intrathoracic pressure, decreases venous return especially in those patients with reduced ejection fraction and heart failure. Increase of intrathoracic pressure, decreases ventricular afterload. If CPAP is to be used to treat a patient with ARF secondary to pneumonia, physicians should be careful in monitoring the hemodynamic effects and the patient's volume status. If necessary, fluid replacement should be assessed prior to CPAP administration [25, 26].

Effects of Continuous Positive Airway Pressure on the Respiratory System

CPAP, recruits collapsed alveoli and improves gas exchange with healing intrathoracic shunt and ventilation/perfusion rate. PEEP opens the collapsed alveoli during expiration. In this way functional residual capacity and compliance increases and work of breathing decreases.

In a study that is evaluated the effect of CPAP (10 cmH_2O) and CPAP with PSV (10-10 cmH2O), PSV (15-5 cmH_2O) in patients with acute lung injury and pneumonia it was indicated that respiratuar frequency decreased with high inspiratory support; arterial oxygenation improved with 10 cmH_2O PEEP; work of breathing decreased with both PSV modalities except CPAP.

Multiple complications may develop in patients in case of invasive mechanical ventilation (IMV). However non-invasive positive pressure ventilation (NPPV), provides respiratory support without invasive intervention and ratio of complication decreases with NPPV. Increase in patient comfort, maintaining airway defense mechanisms, protecting speech, swallowing without inhibiting effective cough and sputum production, enabling effective removal of increased respiratory secretions and providing air flow to obstructed lung areas can be stated as the superior aspects of NPPV to IMV [27].

Conclusion

Chronic Obstructive Pulmonary Disease (COPD): Patients with respiratory failure due to COPD and pneumonia have a higher success rate and NPPV generally preferred as the first line treatment option [28].

Cardiogenic pulmonary edema: The success rate of NPPV was found to be higher in patients with respiratory failure due to pneumonia with cardiogenic pulmonary edema. It is generally preferred as one of the main treatment options for this patients [28].

Interstitial pneumonia: Patients with interstitial pneumonia and associated acute respiratory failure under invasive mechanical ventilation have an increased risk of ventilator-associated lung injury and ventilator-associated pneumonia. Early administration of NPPV is expected to improve prognosis, and reduce short-term mortality in these patients. However there is insufficient evidence regarding the use of NPPV [29].

Immunocompromised patients: NPPV is recommended as first-line therapy in the treatment of patients with immunodeficiency and acute respiratory failure due to pneumonia [19].

Elderly patients: Patients older than 75 years of age with acute hypercapnic respiratory failure due to pneumomia, NPPV has been shown to reduce the need for intubation and mortality by improving arterial blood gases, shortness of breath and NPPV has been recommended as an alternative therapy for elderly patients [24].

Palliative Care

Pneumonia is often the leading cause of death for end-stage elderly patients. For palliative care, NPPV has been found to be more effective than oxygen therapy in reducing shortness of breath, so NPPV may play a role in the treatment of moderate to severe acute respiratory failure with pneumonia [24].

Adult respiratory distress syndrome, community acquired pneumonia, persistence of impaired arterial oxygenation are the significant and independent predictors of NPPV failure in patients with pneumonia [30]. NPPV may be a clinically useful tool in reducing the risk of intubation and mortality. Mortality will be significantly reduced with clinical protocols that define patients who are more likely to benefit from NPPV. Early detection of patients who will fail in NPPV and immediately switch to invasive mechanical ventilation will improve the prognosis and reduce the mortality rate of patients with ARF and pneumonia.

References

[1] Mandell L. A., Wunderink R. G., Anzueto A., Bartlett J. G., Campbell G. D., Dean N. C., Dowell S. F., File Jr. T. M., Musher D. M., Niederman M. S., Torres A., Whitney, C. G., (2007) Infectious Diseases Society of America/American Thoracic

Society consensus guidelines on the management of community-acquired pneumonia in adults. *Clin Infect Dis* 44(Suppl 2):S27–S72.

[2] Restrepo M. I., Anzueto A. (2009) Severe community-acquired pneumonia. *Infect Dis Clin North Am.* 2009 Sep;23(3):503-20. doi: https://doi.org/10.1016/j.idc.2009.04.003.

[3] Levison M. E. Pneumonia, Including Necrotizing Pulmonary Infections (Lung Abscess). In: Braunwald E., Fauci A. S., Hauser S. L., Longo D. L., Kasper D. L., Jameson J. L., editors. *Harrison's Principles of Internal Medicine.* 15th ed. New York: McGraw-Hill; 2001. p. 1475–84.

[4] Hippocrates. *The Genuine Works of Hippocrates,* 1:324. In*: Translated from the Greek with a Preliminary Discourse and Annotations* by Francis Adams. London: Sydenham Society; 1849.

[5] Laennec R. T. *A Treatise on the Diseases of the Chest and on Mediate Auscultation.* In: *Translated from the 3rd French* ed. by J. Forbes, with notes of Prof. Andral from the 4th ed. New York: SS & Wm. Wood; 1838.

[6] Rokitansky C. Inflammations of the lungs (pneumoniae). In: *Manual of Pathological Anatomy.* London: Sydenham Society; 1852.

[7] Sharma S., Maycher, Bruce., Eschun, Gregg. Radiological imaging in pneumonia: recent innovations. *Current Opinion in Pulmonary Medicine,* 2007, 13.3: 159-169.

[8] Kantor H. G. The many radiologic facies of pneumococcal pneumonia. *Am J Roentgenol.* 1981 Dec;137(6):1213-20. doi: https://doi.org/10.2214/ajr.137.6.1213.

[9] Karim R., Andersson, K., Hossain, M. S., Uddin, Md. J., Meah, Md. P. A belief rule based expert system to assess clinical bronchopneumonia suspicion. In: *2016 Future Technologies Conference (FTC).* IEEE, 2016. p. 655-660.

[10] Cottin V., Cordier, Jean-François. Cryptogenic organizing pneumonia. In: Seminars in respiratory and critical care medicine. *Thieme Medical Publishers,* 2012. p. 462-475.

[11] Abbas A. K., Kumar, Vinay, Aster, Jon, C., Robbins Basic Pathology: with student consult Online Access, 9e. 2007. Huang, Chaolin, Wang, Yeming, Li, Xingwang, Ren, Lili, Zhao, Jianping, Hu, Yi, Zhang, Li, Fan, Guohui, Xu, Jiuyang, gu, Xiaoying, Cheng, Zhenshun, Yu, Ting, Xia, Jiaan, Wei, Yuan, Wu, Wenjuan, Xie, Xuelei, Yin, Wen, Li, Hui, Liu, M., Xiao, Yan, Gao, Hong, Guo, Li, Xie, Jungang, Wang, Guangfa, Jiang, Rongmeng, Gao, Zhancheng, Jin, Qi, Wang, Kianwei, Cao, Bin. Clinical features of patients infected with 2019 novel coronavirus in Wuhan, China. *The Lancet,* 2020, 395.10223: 497-506.

[12] Wu Y. C., Chen, Ching-Sung; CHAN, Yu-Jiun. The outbreak of COVID-19: an overview. *Journal of the Chinese Medical Association,* 2020, 83.3: 217.

[13] Meersseman W., Lagrou, Katrien, Maertens, Johan, Wijngaerden, Eric Van. Invasive aspergillosis in the intensive care unit. *Clinical Infectious Diseases,* 2007, 45.2: 205-216.

[14] Marik P. E. Pulmonary aspiration syndromes. *Current Opinion in Pulmonary Medicine,* 2011, 17.3: 148-154.

[15] Diehr, P., R. W. Wood, J. Bushyhead, L. Krueger, B. Wolcott, R. K. Tompkins. Prediction of pneumonia in outpatients with acute cough - a statistical approach. *Journal of Chronic Diseases,* 1984, 37.3: 215-225.

[16] Cunha B. A. The atypical pneumonias: clinical diagnosis and importance. *Clinical Microbiology and Infection*, 2006, 12: 12-24.

[17] Ishiguro T., Noboru Takayanagi, Shozaburo Yamaguchi, Hideaki Yamakawa, Keitaro Nakamoto, Yotaro Takaku, Yosuke Miyahara, Naho Kagiyama, Kazuyoshi Kurashima, Tsutomu Yanagisawa, Yutaka Sugita. Etiology and factors contributing to the severity and mortality of community-acquired pneumonia. *Internal Medicine*, 2013, 52.3: 317-324.

[18] *Mandell's Principles and Practices of Infection Diseases6th Edition* (2004) by Gerald L. Mandell MD, John E. Bennett, Raphael Dolin and Martin J. Blaser. MACP, ISBN 0-443-06643-4 Hardback 4016 Pages Churchill Livingstone.

[19] Fishman J. A., Rubin, Robert H. Infection in organ-transplant recipients. *New England Journal of Medicine,* 1998, 338.24: 1741-1751.

[20] Woodhead, M., F. Blasi, S. Ewig, J. Garau, G. Huchon, M. Ieven, A. Ortqvist, T. Schaberg, A. Torres, G. van der Heijden, R. Read, T. J. M. Verheij. Guidelines for the management of adult lower respiratory tract infections. *European Respiratory Journal*, 2005, 26.6: 1138-1180.

[21] Marik P. E. Aspiration pneumonitis and aspiration pneumonia. *N Engl J Med* 2001;344: 665-71.

[22] DiBardino D. M., Wunderink R. G. Aspiration pneumonia: a review of modern trends. *J Crit Care* 2015; 30: 40-8.

[23] Gleeson K., Eggli D. F., Maxwell S. L. Quantitative aspiration during sleep in normal subjects. *Chest* 1997; 111: 1266-72.

[24] Schmidt-Ioanas M., Lode, Hartmut. Treatment of pneumonia in elderly patients. *Expert Opinion on Pharmacotherapy*, 2006, 7.5: 499-507.

[25] Lenique F., Habis M., Lofaso F., J. L. Dubois-Randé, A. Harf, L. Brochard. Ventilatory and hemodynamic effects of continuous positive airway pressure in left heart failure. *Am J Respir Crit Care Med* 1997;155:500–5.

[26] Rasanen J., Vaisanen I. T., Heikkila J., Nikki P. Acute myocardial infarction complicated by left ventricular dysfunction and respiratory failure. The effects of continuous positive airway pressure. *Chest* 1985;87:158–62.

[27] L'Her E., Deye N., Lellouche F., Solenne Taille, Alexandre Demoule, Amanda Fraticelli, Jordi Mancebo, Laurent Brochard. Physiologic effects of noninvasive ventilation during acute lung injury. *Am J Respir Crit Care Med* 2005;172:1112–8.

[28] Confalonieri M., Potena A., Carbone G., R. D. Porta, E. A. Tolley, G. Umberto Meduri. Acute respiratory failure in patients with severe com- munity-acquired pneumonia: a prospective randomized evaluation of noninvasive ventilation. *Am J Respir Crit Care Med* 1999;160:1585-91.

[29] Visscher D. W., Myers, Jeffrey L. Histologic spectrum of idiopathic interstitial pneumonias. *Proceedings of the American Thoracic Society,* 2006, 3.4: 322-329.

[30] Zhu G. F. Wang D. J. Liu S. Jia M. Jia S. J. Efficacy and safety of noninvasive positive pressure ventilation in the treatment of acute respiratory failure after cardiac surgery. *Chin Med J* (Engl) 2013;126:4463–9.

Chapter 12

Acute Hypoxemic Respiratory Failure Due to COVID-19

Aylin Ozsancak Ugurlu*, **MD**

Department of Pulmonary Medicine, Baskent University, Istanbul, Turkey

Abstract

Acute hypoxemic respiratory failure (ARF) is a characteristic finding of severe COVID-19 pneumonia. Management strategies evolved throughout the pandemic. Non-invasive respiratory support (NIRS) techniques, including high-flow nasal cannula, continuous positive airway pressure and non-invasive ventilation, have been increasingly used in this scenario to prevent unnecessary intubation and protect from its consequences, and to use ICU beds and ventilators effectively.

The response to these strategies can be dependent on patient characteristics (age, comorbidities, severity of the critical illness, etc.) as well as the resources (experience of the health care staff, resource availability.). Main concerns regarding to utilization of NIRS for COVID-19 associated ARF are the risk of viral spreading and delayed intubation leading to increased mortality.

Herein, we reviewed the pathophysiology of COVID-19 associated ARF and accordingly used NIRS strategies, their advantages and disadvantages compared to each other and early intubation, timing of initiation, choice of NIRS, algorithm for selection/combination/switch, monitorization and predictors of NIRS failure.

Keywords: COVID-19, acute hypoxemic respiratory failure, non-invasive ventilation, high-flow oxygen therapy, CPAP

---

* Corresponding Author's Email: aozsancak@hotmail.com.

In: Nasal High Flow and Non-Invasive Ventilatory Support
Editors: A. M. Esquinas, D. A. Lagonidis, P. Silva Santos et al.
ISBN: 979-8-88697-420-1

Introduction

Coronavirus disease 2019 (COVID-19) is an evolving disease with a wide spectrum of clinical features, ranging from asymptomatic to critical illness and even death. As of Feb 25th, 2022, 430 million cases of COVID-19 and approximately 6 million deaths were reported all over the world [1]. Acute hypoxemic respiratory failure (ARF) is the characteristic finding of severe COVID-19 and requires oxygen and ventilatory support. Once oxygen requirements increase, non-invasive respiratory support, including continuous positive airway pressure (CPAP), bilevel positive airway pressure (NIV) and high-flow nasal cannula (HFNC) has been commonly used to prevent the significant mortality and morbidity associated with invasive mechanical ventilation (IMV). NIRS has also assisted in effective use of limited ICU beds and ventilators.

In this chapter, we will discuss the basic pathophysiology of ARF in COVID-19, the types of NIRS, timing and appropriate use of NIRS, comparison of NIRS-related outcomes, monitorization and predictors of failure.

Pathophysiology of COVID-19-Related and Non-Invasive Support

The pathophysiology of ARF due to COVID-19 pneumonia is peculiar. In COVID-associated ARDS (cARDS); prevalent interstitial and microvascular involvement, leading to development of lung injury, is followed by a more classic picture of diffuse alveolar damage with hyaline membrane formation, edema, and fibrotic deposition, similar to classical ARDS [2]. In the *L phenotype* (low elastance, low lung weight, and low recruitability), the hypoxic vasoconstriction mechanism is disrupted, due to the inflammatory storm and the appearance of microthrombi, and eventually ventilation-perfusion mismatch develops [3]. The pulmonary mechanics are preserved, which can be related to less dyspnea than expected for that level of severe hypoxemia, known as '*silent/happy hypoxemia.*'

Another explanation for this decreased dyspnea can be the presence of right-left intrapulmonary shunt inducing hypoxemia with increase in minute ventilation and subsequent hypocapnia [3]. The *H phenotype* (high elastance, high recruitability), commonly observed in the later stage of the disease, is similar to classical ARDS. In this case, respiratory mechanics is impaired with increased $PaCO_2$.

The clinical and epidemiological features of COVID-19 are understood, however discussions about management still continue. Clinicians can direct the treatment by considering the pathophysiology in the current situation. For example, in the first phase, the progressive escalation of oxygen therapy may be more suitable management strategy instead of alveolar recruitment with positive pressure, which would better be reserved for later phase.

However, the use of NIRS, especially NIV, is still controversial in this scenario [4]. The application of pressure support in a spontaneously breathing patient with tachypnea and high tidal volume may result in excessive negative intrathoracic pressure fluctuations, and subsequently *self-induced lung injury (P-SILI)*. It can be also due to in-homogeneity in gas distribution and changes in pulmonary perfusion [3]. Besides, the utilization of NIRS may delay intubation, with increased risk of mortality. On the other hand, NIRS techniques can avoid unnecessary intubations and associated consequences and mortality, especially during pandemics with exponential growth of admitted patients, shortage of ICU beds and ventilators. Additionally, CPAP can reduce the risk for P-SILI with application of same level of positive airway pressure as compared to NIV and can also favor the redistribution of perfusion to newly recruited depending on areas in first phase.

At the beginning of the pandemic, *early intubation* was recommended since the success rate (i.e., avoidance of intubation and in-hospital death) of NIV or CPAP was low (<1/3) [5, 6]. It was also suggested to protect health-care workers from cross infections via aerosol formation, especially during NIV with oronasal mask or HFNC use. While most of the critically ill patients were intubated early in New York, China preferred NIRS over IMV [7]. However, the success rates increased (to 70%) with the organization of dedicated units with appropriate staff, monitoring and patient selection, as well as increasing use of adjunct therapies including corticosteroids [6], evolving the current management into a more non-invasive pathway. As a result, use of IMV decreased leading to a parallel reduction in length of ICU stay and in-hospital mortality during 2nd wave compared to 1st wave [8]. In a recent meta-analysis suggested that timing of intubation (early vs. late) may have no effect on mortality and morbidity of critically ill patients with COVID-19, justifying a wait-and-see approach, with possible fewer intubations [9].

One of the greatest concerns during application of NIRS modalities in COVID-19-associated ARF is the risk of viral transmission. Based on current literature, the exact amount to which HFNC or NIV expose healthcare workers to viral transmission is unknown, but it does not seem to differ significantly than spontaneous breathing or COT [10]. It can be suggested that fewer droplets are spread with the helmet. In other devices, both the structural features of the device and the pressures/flow used can increase droplet dispersion. In all cases, measures such as well ventilation of the rooms, providing a negative pressure system, covering the devices with masks, keeping the positive pressure support or flow at the lowest possible value, and fitting the mask tight enough to avoid leakage are necessary to prevent viral spreading.

Therefore, each phase requires individualized management approach, in terms of oxygenation and positive pressure application. NIRS is primarily considered if it provides correction of hypoxemia and reduction of inspiratory effort. However, in ineffective cases with NIRS, mechanical ventilation should be considered without delay to ensure oxygenation and prevent P-SILI (Figure 1).

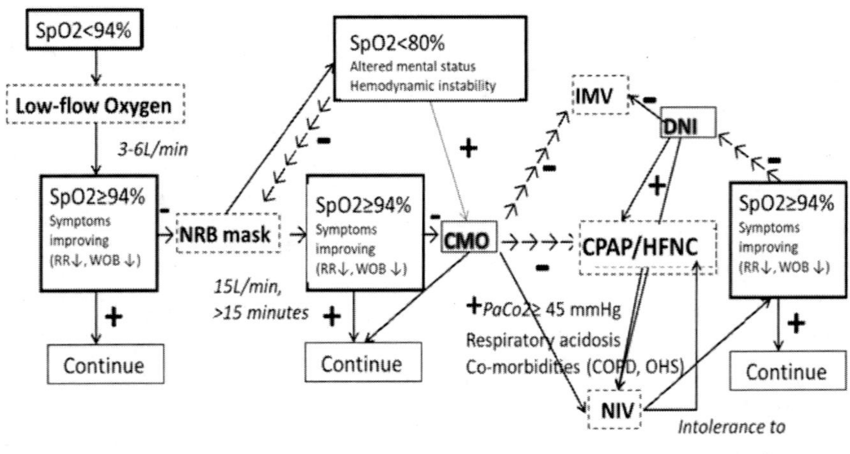

CMO: comfort measures only; CPAP: continuous positive airway pressure; DNI: do-not-intubate; HFNC: high flow nasal cannula; IMV: invasive mechanical ventilation; NIV: non-invasive ventilation; NRB: non re-breather; SpO_2: oxygen saturation.

Figure 1. Algorithm for NIRS use.

Options: Non-Invasive Respiratory Support

The most commonly used NIRS strategies in this scenario are HFNC, CPAP and NIV [7, 8] (Table 1). The *HFNC* can provide gas flows that match the patient's average inspiratory flow generated by the high respiratory drive. Thus, oxygen can be supplied to the patient at the adjusted FiO_2. The additional benefits of dead space washout, air warming and humidification can contribute to reducing airway resistance and respiratory effort. However, its application via two nasal prongs without a tight fitting seal around the patient's face can increase the risk of aerosolization. It is generally started with a flow of 30 L/min titrated up to 60 L/min, and FiO_2 up to 100%, to keep oxygen saturation >93% [11].

Table 1. Advantages and disadvantages of NIRS strategies

	Advantages	Disadvantages
HFNC	• Easy application and delivery • Potential to free up ventilators in regions struggling with ventilator shortages • Increased patient comfort • Better tolerance • Improved airway clearance • Reduced upper airway space • Provision of low PEEP (up to 7 cmH2O) • Does not induce alveolar over distension	• Risk of viral spreading (especially with higher flows) • Need to use large amounts of oxygen • A true PEEP effect cannot be achieved • Low PEEP and supra-physiological FiO2 leading to resorption atelectasis • Not easy to monitor VT and MV, with increased risk of P-SILI
CPAP/NIV	• Decreased risk of viral spreading with tightly fitted helmet or oronasal mask, double circuit, and antimicrobial filter • Increase resistance in the small vessels of non-dependent regions of the lung, favoring the redistribution of perfusion to newly recruited depending on areas • Reduce the respiratory work and distress • The graphical monitoring of ventilator parameters, flow, and pressure waveforms	• Less comfortable and less tolerated. • Requires more experienced staff and their time • Risk of generating excessive negative intra-thoracic pressure fluctuations • Risk of viral spreading with nasal pillows or with mask leakage

MV, minute ventilation; PEEP, positive end-expiratory pressure; P-SILI, self –induced lung injury; VT, tidal volume.

CPAP application provides a single level of positive airway pressure throughout the breathing cycle; thus, it can recruit non-aerated alveoli in dependent pulmonary regions, improve arterial oxygenation (especially in edema and atelectasis) and reduce respiratory work. It is generally started with 10 cmH_2O (not exceeding 12-13 cmH_2O to prevent P-SILI), pressure and FiO_2 are titrated to achieve target oxygen saturation >93% or PaO_2 > 60% [11]. *NIV* provides additional inspiratory pressure support. NIV can increase alveolar ventilation and reduce the workload of respiratory muscles. Especially, in hypoxemia-associated with deterioration in ventilation mechanics, it is most administered as bilevel positive airway pressure and generally preferred in patients with co-morbid conditions with hypercapnia, such as COPD, obesity-hypoventilation syndrome [7, 11]. The use of helmet or oronasal mask tightly fitted on patient, with double circuit and antimicrobial filter, can decrease the risk of aerosolization [10]. PEEP of 12-16 cmH_2O and pressure support set with the aim of tidal volume of 4-6 ml/kg and FiO_2 aim of target oxygen saturation 90-95% are recommended [11].

When to Start?

When conventional oxygen therapy is insufficient to provide the required oxygenation, it should be switched to one of the appropriate NIRS techniques. Preference should be made considering the complications of invasive ventilation and intubation, and whether NIRS techniques will be sufficient, and more importantly, the possibility of increasing self-injury in patients whose efforts in spontaneous ventilation with NIRS continue. Proper timing for NIRS can prevent self-injury [3]. Although the recommendations at the beginning of the pandemic were generally based on old experiences, the new recommendations have been made as the experience of COVID-19 and ARF increased [3].

With the early Italian triage, four categories were determined according to SaO_2, respiratory rate and oxygen response. In a multicenter study with this classification, the indication for starting NIV corresponded to the third (orange) category ($SaO_2 < 94\%$, RR > 20 but poor response to 10–15 L/min oxygen and requiring CPAP/NIV with very high FiO_2). Winck et al., proposed two different scenarios for starting NIRS: *Early start* (PaO_2: $FiO_2 < 300$ or $SpO_2 < 93\%$ on $O_2 > 5$ L/min or $SpO_2 < 94\%$ with FiO_2 40%) or *late start* ($SpO_2 < 92\%$ under O_2 at 15 L/min or $PaO_2/FiO_2 < 150$) [11]. They suggested that the PaO_2/FiO_2 index may not reflect the severity of the exchange, as it does not consider the baseline $PaCO_2$ value, which is usually decreased in patients with ARF secondary to COVID-19.

Guideline recommendations have varied widely [3, 7, 11, 14]. The heterogeneity in NIRS initiation criteria has also been evident in the only 2 RCT's done in this field, including Respiratory Support (RS)-RECOVERY [12] and HENIVOT [13] with a $FiO_2 \geq 40\%$ and a peripheral $SpO_2 \leq 94\%$, and a sole criterion of PaO_2/FiO_2 of <200, respectively.

Which Modality to Choose?

In COVID-19 pandemic, the use of any modality of NIRS has been generally driven by the primary physician's discretion and has varied greatly depending on changes in practice over time, as well as on geographical region, hospital, clinicians, and resource limitations. The current international guidelines vary widely concerning the optimal NIRS for patients with COVID-19-related hypoxemia, reflecting the lack of large-scale randomized control trials in this field [12, 13]. While most of the experts suggested HFNC as the first-line strategy as NIRS, others recommended CPAP/NIV especially with helmet interface [3, 7, 11, 14].

HFNC can be considered an alternative strategy for oxygen supplementation prior to IMV and should be used in patients unable to maintain $SpO_2 > 90\%$ or may be used in patients with increasing oxygen requirements [3]. (Figure 1). It was shown to be used between 23-64% of patients with severe COVID-19 pneumonia worldwide [8]. Positive pressure devices (*CPAP, NIV*), as other options for NIRS, can prevent alveolar collapse by providing expiratory positive pressure support, reduce ventilation/ perfusion mismatch and improve gas exchange. Therefore, NIV has been especially recommended in case of hypercapnic respiratory failure with respiratory acidosis and increased work of breathing.

On the other hand, CPAP has been used more than NIV outside the ICU [8], since it is easier to apply outside ICU, requires less expertise from personnel compared to NIV and can be delivered with simpler devices. It may also be necessary to escalate the treatment or to combine it with other modalities, depending on the course of the disease and follow-up findings. There are also opinions advocating switching to direct IMV in case of failure with NIRS, while NIV is recommended to provide positive pressure support in HFNC failure. Awake proning and the semi-prone position (Rodin's thinker) can also be combined to NIRS strategies to improve oxygenation.

In a recent meta-analysis regarding NIRS use in pandemic8, including 13,931 patients from 22 prospective and 61 retrospective observational studies, as well as 2 RCT's [12, 13]; CPAP was the most commonly used 'sole modality,' followed by HFNC and NIV. In some cases, patients escalated from HFNC to CPAP or NIV to provide increased respiratory support, while in others vice versa because intolerance to mask, hood, or device. Intubation was prevented in 61% of the 12,633 patients receiving NIRS, depending on the patient demographics (age and co-morbidities), baseline severity of respiratory and other organ dysfunction, DNI status, degree of systemic inflammation, and response to a trial of NIRS. Overall survival was 66%, while it was 30% for patients with do-not-intubate (DNI) order. CPAP was more commonly used as a ceiling of treatment. For patients without DNI order, survival was similar among NIRS modalities. In one of the studies [15] including 670 patients, intubation rate was similar between 3 forms of NIRS.

In Italian randomized study [13], HFNC and NIV with helmet interface were compared. Although the intubation rate and days without IMV were significantly lower in the NIV group, there was no difference in hospital mortality. In the other RCT from UK comparing 3 NIRS modalities [12]; while no difference was observed in the use of HFNC compared to COT, the need for intubation and mortality as a composite outcome were found to be lower in the CPAP group compared to COT.

Monitorization

To protect from increased risk of delayed intubation, as the second important concern regarding to NIRS management; it is important to closely monitor patients to evaluate their response to NIRS modality. The treatment can continue in the same way, switch to a different NIRS modality, or progress to intubation based on assessment [3]. (Figure 1). In order to standardize this evaluation, various indexes/scores have been studied.

An increase in *ROX index* [i.e., (SpO_2/FiO_2):RR], especially in patients who received HFNC, was shown to be associated with recovery in patients receiving HFOT due to COVID-related ARF [3, 6, 8, 11]. In positive pressure therapies, PaO_2/FiO_2, alveolo-arterial gradient or HACOR score (heart rate, acidosis, consciousness level, oxygenation, respiratory rate), as well as clinical improvement and hemodynamic tolerance can be followed-up to monitor the response. Additionally, tidal volume can be tracked after, specifically to prevent P-SILI.

Predictors of Failure

A variety of risk factors for NIRS failure was described by 54 papers, including older age; presence, number, or type of co-morbidities; illness severity on admission to hospital or ICU; worse oxygenation on admission to hospital; worse respiratory function before NIRS; poor response in respiratory variables to NIRS over 1-6 hours; higher circulating concentration of C-reactive protein [8]. Additionally, it can be related to NIRS initiation criteria, the interface used, the protocols used by the center, the basic monitoring capacity, and the education level of the team. Differences in the results of the studies may also be due to these discrepancies.

Early detection of treatment failure in these patients, evaluation of the necessity for intubation in case of no clinical improvement or worsening in 48-72 hours of NIRS treatment may have a positive effect on mortality.

Conclusion

The utilization of NIRS strategies for ARF, associated with COVID-19 requiring additional ventilator support to COT, can reduce the mortality rates and consequences associated with early intubation. Large-scale research is still needed to determine the best algorithm for escalation of NIRS modalities.

References

[1] *WHO Coronavirus (COVID-19) Dashboard.* https://covid19.who.int/. Accessed by February 25th, 2022.

[2] Gattinoni L., Coppola S., Cressoni M., Busana M., Rossi S., Chiumello D. COVID-19 Does Not Lead to a "Typical" Acute Respiratory Distress Syndrome. *Am J Respir Crit Care Med.* 2020; 201: 1299-1300.

[3] Luján M., Sayas J., Mediano O., Egea C. Non-invasive Respiratory Support in COVID-19: A Narrative Review. *Front Med (Lausanne).* 2022 Jan 4; 8: 788190.

[4] Cosentini R., Groff P., Brambilla A. M., Camajori Todeschini R., Gangitano G., Ingrassia S., Marino R., Nori F., Pagnozzi F., Panero F., Ferrari R. SIMEU NIV Group collaborators. SIMEU position paper on non-invasive respiratory support in COVID-19 pneumonia. *Intern Emerg Med.* 2022 Feb 1:1–15.

[5] Zuo M. Z., Huang Y. G., Ma W. H., Xue Z. G., Zhang J. Q., Gong Y. H., Che L. Chinese Society of Anesthesiology Task Force on Airway Management, Airway Management Chinese Society of Anesthesiology Task Force on. Expert Recommendations for Tracheal Intubation in Critically ill Patients with Noval Coronavirus Disease 2019. *Chin Med Sci J.* 2020;35(2):105–9.

[6] Groff P., Ferrari R. Non-invasive respiratory support in the treatment of acute hypoxemic respiratory failure secondary to COVID-19 related pneumonia. *Eur J Intern Med.* 2021 Apr;86:17-21.

[7] Sullivan Z. P., Zazzeron L., Berra L., Hess D. R., Bittner E. A., Chang M. G. Noninvasive respiratory support for COVID-19 patients: when, for whom, and how? *J Intensive Care.* 2022 Jan 15;10(1):3.

[8] Weerakkody S., Arina P, Glenister J., Cottrell S., Boscaini-Gilroy G., Singer M., Montgomery H. E. Considerations for clinical practice and priorities for research. *Lancet Respir Med.* 2022;10(2):199-213.

[9] Papoutsi E., Giannakoulis V. G., Xourgia E., Routsi C., Kotanidou A., Siempos I. I. Effect of timing of intubation on clinical outcomes of critically ill patients with COVID-19: a systematic review and meta-analysis of non-randomized cohort studies. *Crit Care.* 2021;25(1):121.

[10] Oliveira M. R., Back G. D., de Mello Konzen V., Garcia-Araújo A. S., da Luz Goulart C., Nunes Silva R., Mara Wibelinger L., Dixit S., Arena R., Borghi-Silva A. Noninvasive ventilation in patients with COVID-19 from the perspective of the risk of contamination: a narrative review. *Expert Rev Respir Med.* 2022 Jan;16(1):67-77.

[11] Winck J. C., Scala R. Non-invasive respiratory support paths in hospitalized patients with COVID-19: proposal of an algorithm. *Pulmonology.* 2021 Jul-Aug;27(4):305-312.

[12] Perkins G. D., Ji C, Connolly B. A., Couper K., Lall R., Baillie J. K., Bradley J. M., Dark P., Dave C., De Soyza A., Dennis A. V., Devrell A., Fairbairn S., Ghani H., Gorman E. A., Green C. A., Hart N., Hee S. W., Kimbley Z., Madathil S., McGowan N., Messer B., Naisbitt J., Norman C., Parekh D., Parkin E. M., Patel J., Regan S. E., Ross C., Rostron A. J., Saim M., Simonds A. K., Skilton E., Stallard N., Steiner M., Vancheeswaran R., Yeung J., McAuley D. F. RECOVERY-RS Collaborators. Effect of Noninvasive Respiratory Strategies on Intubation or Mortality Among Patients with Acute Hypoxemic Respiratory Failure and COVID-19: The RECOVERY-RS Randomized Clinical Trial. *JAMA.* 2022;327(6):546-558.

[13] Grieco D. L., Menga L. S., Cesarano M., Rosà T., Spadaro S., Bitondo M. M., Montomoli J., Falò G., Tonetti T., Cutuli S. L., Pintaudi G., Tanzarella E. S., Piervincenzi E., Bongiovanni F., Dell'Anna A. M., Delle Cese L., Berardi C., Carelli S., Bocci M. G., Montini L., Bello G., Natalini D., De Pascale G., Velardo M., Volta C. A., Ranieri V. M., Conti G., Maggiore S. M., Antonelli M., COVID-ICU Gemelli Study Group. Effect of Helmet Noninvasive Ventilation vs. High-Flow Nasal Oxygen on Days Free of Respiratory Support in Patients With COVID-19 and Moderate to Severe Hypoxemic Respiratory Failure: The HENIVOT Randomized Clinical Trial. *JAMA.* 2021; 325(17):1731-1743.

[14] Akoumianaki E., Ischaki E., Karagiannis K., Sigala I., Zakyn-Thinos S. The Role of Noninvasive Respiratory Management in Patients with Severe COVID-19 Pneumonia. *J Pers Med.* 2021;11(9):884.

[15] Franco C., Facciolongo N., Tonelli R., Dongilli R., Vianello A., Pisani L., Scala R., Malerba M., Carlucci A., Negri E. A., Spoladore G., Arcaro G., Tillio P. A., Lastoria C., Schifino G., Tabbì L., Guidelli L., Guaraldi G., Ranieri V. M., Clini E., Nava S. Feasibility and clinical impact of out-of-ICU noninvasive respiratory support in patients with COVID-19-related pneumonia. *Eur Respir J.* 2020;56(5):2002130.

Chapter 13

Respiratory Failure in Acute Heart Failure

Stefano Oldani[1,*], MD
Andrea De Vito[2], MD
Serena Bensai[1], MD
and Lara Bertolovic[1], MD

[1] Department of Thoracic Diseases, Pulmonary Operative Unit,
Morgagni Pierantoni Hospital, Health Local Agency of Romagna, Forlì, Italy
[2] Head and Neck Department, ENT Unit, Ravenna - Lugo Hospitals,
Health Local Agency of Romagna, Ravenna, Italy

Abstract

Acute heart failure (AHF) is a rapid or gradual onset of symptoms and signs of heart failure that, in the more severe scenario, can present as cardiogenic pulmonary edema (CPE) or cardiogenic shock. A rapid assessment of the patient is crucial to improve survival. Initial management requires aggressive pharmacologic treatment with loop diuretics and sometimes vasodilators or inotropic agents.

If acute respiratory failure occurs, the patient must be supported according to his/her need with conventional oxygen therapy (COT), high-flow nasal cannulae (HFNC), positive airway pressure (PAP) therapies or invasive mechanical ventilation (IMV). PAP therapies have shown some favorable effects on blood oxygenation and on patients' hemodynamics. In fact, PAP therapies may achieve a reduction of right ventricle (RV) preload, a potential increase of pulmonary vascular resistance (PVR) and a reduction of left ventricle (LV) transmural pressure gradient, hence reducing LV afterload and stroke work.

---

* Corresponding Author's Email: stefano.oldani11289@gmail.com.

In: Nasal High Flow and Non-Invasive Ventilatory Support
Editors: A. M. Esquinas, D. A. Lagonidis, P. Silva Santos et al.
ISBN: 979-8-88697-420-1

Keywords: cardiogenic pulmonary edema, acute respiratory failure, heart lung interactions, continuous positive pressure ventilation (CPAP), non-invasive ventilation (NIV)

Introduction

Acute hearth failure (AHF) is a rapid or gradual onset of symptoms and signs of heart failure severe enough for the patient to seek urgent medical attention. Its clinical features are breathlessness, ankle swelling, fatigue, along with pulmonary crackles and elevated jugular venous pressure. This condition is a leading cause of hospital admission especially in the elderly and it is associated with high in-hospital mortality (4-10%) and rehospitalization rates.

AHF can also present as acute cardiogenic pulmonary edema (CPE), a life-threatening cause of acute respiratory failure (ARF), that can potentially lead to hemodynamic instability and cardiogenic shock. CPE presents with rapidly worsening dyspnea, due to accumulation of fluid within the lung's interstitial and alveolar space, that results from an acute elevation in cardiac filling pressures.

AHF can be the first manifestation of HF, but it is usually caused by a decompensation of an underlying chronic heart failure (CHF), resulting from systolic and/or diastolic disfunction of the LV, valvular diseases, or coronary artery disease [1].

Several conditions can rapidly precipitate an AHF. These precipitating factors can be categorized as [2]:

- *Causes of increased preload*: volume overload (such as saline infusion or blood transfusion) or acute aortic or mitral regurgitation.
- *Causes of decreased cardiac contractility*: usually myocadiac ischemia/infarction.
- *Causes of increased afterload*: hypertensive crisis or acute obstruction of heart chambers due to intracardiac masses, or thrombosis of mechanical valves.

Initial Management and Pharmacologic Treatment of AHF/CPE

Patients presenting with AHF should be assessed and stabilized swiftly.

The initial approach includes [1]:

- Assessment of vital signs (blood pressure, EKG and SpO2 monitoring).
- Appropriate respiratory assistance, escalating from conventional oxygen therapy to HFNC, CPAP/bilevel NIV or even immediate invasive ventilation.
- Prompt diuretic therapy with loop diuretic drugs.
- Urine output monitoring.

Pharmacologic Treatment

Loop diuretics are important in controlling dyspnea and other symptoms related to fluid overload. In fact, they provide an immediate reduction in the venous tone, followed by an increased diuresis, hence a reduction of LV preload. Moreover, loop diuretics' administration is linked to an improvement of in-hospital mortality [3].

Another optional medical treatment is the administration of vasodilator drugs that can aim to lower the arterial tone (es. nitroprusside) or the venous tone (es. nitroglycerine). The first is recommended in patients who require a rapid decrease of systemic vascular resistance and LV afterload (systolic BP > 110mmHg or acute aortic or mitral regurgitation), whereas the latter is suggested when the initial diuretic therapy is not sufficient to alleviate respiratory distress [4].

Opiates have been widely used during CPE to better control dyspnea. However, there is limited evidence to support their use in this condition. In fact, the largest studies found that morphine was linked to increased need of mechanical ventilation, admission to the ICU and in-hospital mortality [5].

Inotropic agents, such as dobutamine or dopamine, can be used as a temporary measure to support patients with systolic BP < 90mmHg who do not respond to standard treatment, including fluid challenge, to improve peripheral perfusion and maintain end-organ function. However, evidence of safety and efficacy of these treatments is lacking. There are also some concerns that inotropic agents may be detrimental, since they can increase heart rate, risk of arrythmias and myocardial oxygen consumption, thus provoking further ischemia [6, 7].

A vasopressor, preferably noradrenalin, may be considered in patients with cardiogenic shock to increase arterial BP, hereby improving vital organ perfusion [1].

Lastly, thromboembolism prophylaxis with heparin is recommended in patients with no contraindications and not already treated with anticoagulants to reduce the risk of deep venous thrombosis and pulmonary embolism [1].

Supplemental Oxygen and Positive Pressure Therapies (CPAP/Bilevel NIV) in AHF/CPE

Conventional oxygen therapy, i.e., oxygen administration via nasal cannula, venturi-mask or reservoir bag mask, must be provided as soon as acute respiratory failure occurs (SpO_2 <90% or PaO_2 <60mmHg) to achieve an SpO_2 > 90%. As a general precaution, if the patient is at risk of CO_2 retention (e.g., underlying COPD), O_2 administration has to be less aggressive. In fact, a target SpO_2 of 88-92% is acceptable to guarantee an adequate blood oxygenation, avoiding iatrogenic hypercapnia. It is also important to point out that oxygen is not recommended as a routine therapy in patients without hypoxemia, since it may cause vasoconstriction and reduce cardiac output [1].

However, if respiratory distress, respiratory acidosis and/or hypoxemia persist despite COT, a trial with PAP therapies, either CPAP or bilevel NIV, is recommended [1, 8].

The Hemodynamic Consequences of PAP Therapies

There are some important heart-lung interactions during the breathing cycle. To better understand these phenomena, it is important to observe that [9]:

- The heart can be considered a pressure chamber in another pressure chamber, the thorax.
- Changes in intrathoracic pressure are transmitted to the intrathoracic cardiovascular system, depending on the lung and chest wall compliance.
- Lung volumes affect pulmonary vascular resistance (PVR), following a U-shaped curve. The nadir of PVR occurs at functional respiratory capacity.

During spontaneous breathing, a negative intrathoracic pressure is recorded in the inspiratory phase, thus enhancing venous return to the right heart. However, as soon as a positive end expiratory pressure (PEEP) is administered, intrathoracic pressure increases throughout the respiratory cycle, leading to a reduction of venous return along with an increase of the diameter of the inferior vena cava (IVC). It has been shown that cardiac output was reduced by 10% with bilevel ventilation with zero PEEP, 18% with a PEEP of 9cmH_2O and up to 36% with a PEEP of 16cmH_2O [10].

PEEP can also influence the perfusion of the lung vessels. In fact, PEEP can recruit collapsed lung units, possibly reducing PVR and improving blood oxygenation. This reduction in PVR may be due to the re-expansion of previously collapsed areas, thus restoring lung volumes, but also to a reversion of the hypoxic vasoconstriction reflex, typical of non-ventilated areas. However, if lung hyperinflation occurs, such as during a high PEEP ventilation, small lung vessels may be squeezed, increasing PVR and consequently RV afterload. This increase can also cause a reduction of RV output, that can lead to a reduced left heart preload and output. It is therefore possible for PEEP to both raise and lower PVR.

Moreover, systemic circulation can be affected by increased intrathoracic pressure. As aforementioned, a reduction of venous return can lead to a reduced cardiac output, especially in case of hypovolemia.

Nevertheless, PAP therapies can reduce LV stroke work, and, to an extent, this can mitigate the effect of decreased LV preload. In fact, during spontaneous breathing, the negative intrathoracic pressure recorded during the inspiratory phase, especially in patients with an increased work of breathing, can oppose LV contraction, increasing its transmural pressure. When PEEP is applied, these swings in intrathoracic pressure become less wide throughout the respiratory cycle, hence reducing transmural LV pressure and therefore LV afterload and stroke work.

To summarize, during PAP therapies, RV preload is decreased and PVR might be increased, possibly increasing RV afterload. On the other hand, PAP therapies reduce LV transmural pressure gradient, hence reducing LV afterload and stroke work [9].

These beneficial effects require blood pressure to be regularly monitored during PAP therapies, especially in patients with reduced preload reserve (hypovolemia) or hypotension [1].

The Role of PAP Therapies during AHF/CPE

As aforementioned, PAP therapies may be beneficial in AHF/CPE to reduce cardiac preload, prevent alveolar collapse and decrease LV afterload.

In fact, PAP therapies have been shown to improve mortality, need for intubation and clinical and laboratory signs of respiratory failure (e.g., heart rate, dyspnea, hypercapnia and respiratory acidosis). However, most metanalysis compare PAP therapies (CPAP or bilevel NIV) with standard medical care alone. Thus, data of superiority of CPAP over NIV or vice versa are limited [11].

For example, one metanalysis showed that CPAP on top of medical therapy was linked to lower hospital mortality when compared with medical therapy alone. On the other hand, the same metanalysis showed that NIV was only associated with a trend towards improved mortality and did not reach statistical significance [12].

However, only one randomized trial compared CPAP with bilevel NIV and found no difference in mortality or intubation rate between the two groups, although respiratory distress appeared to resolve sooner among patients treated with bilevel NIV [13].

There are also some data that suggest that the use of PAP therapies during CPE is linked to an increased risk of new onset myocardial infarction, but evidence in this field is scant. Nevertheless, the aforementioned favorable effect of PAP therapies appears to be greater than this meager risk [1].

Some trials also explore the role of PAP therapies in the pre-hospital care of CPE. These trials are heterogeneous, but the pooled analysis performed in the ERS/ATS guidelines of NIV in ARF, proves that PAP therapies, even in this setting, can further decrease mortality and the need for intubation [8].

Our clinical experience suggests starting with a trial of CPAP via face mask or helmet, since this modality is easier to apply. Moreover, CPAP can also be provided with simpler and cheaper technology (venturimeter with PEEP valve, Boussignac systems, flow generators), that do not even require a ventilator. All these reasons make CPAP more feasible for the emergency setting, especially in the pre-hospital management [8].

We therefore reserve NIV for more severe patients, with respiratory distress despite CPAP, or with acute respiratory acidosis, where CPAP with a high PEEP may be detrimental (e.g., pre-existent COPD, due to the risk of worsening intrinsic-PEEP).

Recently, some clinical trials have explored the role of HFNC in CPE treatment. HFNC has been shown to be superior to COT in ameliorating ABG parameters and respiratory dynamic. Moreover, another pilot study that compared HFNC to bilevel NIV in the treatment of type 2 respiratory failure due to CPE, showed a non-inferiority of the first. This data is compelling, but not sufficient to replace NIV with HFNC in this clinical scenario. However, providing HFNC rather than COT can be reasonable [14, 15].

Nevertheless, hypoxaemia in CPE usually resolves quickly with prompt treatment. Therefore, if hypoxemia persists despite PAP therapies, or if symptoms and sings of cardiac shock occur, endotracheal intubation and invasive ventilation must not be delayed.

Conclusion

AHF is a rapid or gradual onset of symptoms and signs of heart failure that, in the more severe scenario, can present as CPE or cardiogenic shock. Initial management requires assessment of vital signs (blood pressure, EKG and SpO_2 monitoring), appropriate respiratory assistance (COT/HFNC/PAP therapies/IMV), prompt diuretic therapy with loop diuretic drugs, urine output monitoring. As soon as respiratory failure occurs, a trial with COT, or better with HFNC, is recommended. If not sufficient, patients must be rapidly escalated to CPAP or bilevel NIV to reduce mortality and the need of intubation.

During PAP therapies, RV preload is decreased and PVR might be increased, possibly increasing RV afterload. On the other hand, PAP therapies reduce LV transmural pressure gradient, hence reducing LV afterload and stroke work. Respiratory failure due to CPE usually resolves quickly. Therefore, if hypoxemia persists despite PAP therapies, or if symptoms and signs of cardiac shock occur, endotracheal intubation and invasive ventilation must not be delayed.

References

[1] McDonagh, T. A., Metra, M., Adamo, M., Gardner, R. S., Baumbach, A., Böhm, et al. 2021 ESC Guidelines for the diagnosis and treatment of acute and chronic heart failure. *Eur. Heart J.* 2021, 42, 3599–3726.

[2] Heart Failure Society of America. HFSA 2010 Comprehensive Heart Failure Practice Guideline. *J. Card. Fail.* 2010, 16, e1–e2.

[3] Felker, G. M., Ellison, D. H., Mullens, W., Cox, Z. L. & Testani, J. M. Diuretic Therapy for Patients With Heart Failure. *J. Am. Coll. Cardiol.* 2020, 75, 1178–1195.

[4] Kozhuharov, N., Goudev, A., Flores, D., Maeder, M. T., Walter, J., Shrestha, S., et al. Effect of a Strategy of Comprehensive Vasodilation vs Usual Care on Mortality and Heart Failure Rehospitalization Among Patients With Acute Heart Failure. *JAMA* 2019, 322, 2292.

[5] Peacock, W. F., Hollander, J. E., Diercks, D. B., Lopatin, M., Fonarow, G. & Emerman, C. L. Morphine and outcomes in acute decompensated heart failure: an ADHERE analysis. *Emerg. Med. J.* 2008, 25, 205–209.

[6] Abraham, W. T., Adams, K. F., Fonarow, G. C., Costanzo, M. R., Berkowitz, R. L., LeJemtel, T. H., Cheng, M. L. & Wynne, J. In-Hospital Mortality in Patients With Acute Decompensated Heart Failure Requiring Intravenous Vasoactive Medications. *J. Am. Coll. Cardiol.* 2005, 46, 57–64.

[7] Burger, A. J., Elkayam, U., Neibaur, M. T., Haught, H., Ghali, J., Horton, D. P. & Aronson, D. Comparison of the occurrence of ventricular arrhythmias in patients with acutely decompensated congestive heart failure receiving dobutamine versus nesiritide therapy. *Am. J. Cardiol.* 2001, 88, 35–39.

[8] Rochwerg, B., Brochard, L., Elliott, M. W., Hess, D., Hill, N. S., Nava, S., Navalesi, P., Antonelli, M., Brozek, J., Conti, G., Ferrer, M., Guntupalli, K., Jaber, S., Keenan, S., Mancebo, J., Mehta, S. & Raoof, S. Official ERS/ATS clinical practice guidelines: noninvasive ventilation for acute respiratory failure. *Eur. Respir. J.* 2017, 50, 1602426.

[9] Corp, A., Thomas, C. & Adlam, M. The cardiovascular effects of positive pressure ventilation. *BJA Educ.* 2021, 21, 202–209.

[10] Berglund, J. E., Haldén, E., Jakobson, S. & Landelius, J. Echocardiographic analysis of cardiac function during high PEEP ventilation. *Intensive Care Med.* 1994, 20, 174–180.

[11] Berbenetz, N., Wang, Y., Brown, J., Godfrey, C., Ahmad, M., Vital, F. M., Lambiase, P., Banerjee, A., Bakhai, A. & Chong, M. Non-invasive positive pressure ventilation (CPAP or bilevel NPPV) for cardiogenic pulmonary oedema. *Cochrane Database Syst. Rev.* 2019, doi:10.1002/14651858.CD005351.pub4.

[12] Gray, A., Goodacre, S., Newby, D. E., Masson, M., Sampson, F. & Nicholl, J. Noninvasive Ventilation in Acute Cardiogenic Pulmonary Edema. *N. Engl. J. Med.* 2008, 359, 142–151.

[13] Nouira, S., Boukef, R., Bouida, W., Kerkeni, W., Beltaief, K., Boubaker, H., Boudhib, L., Grissa, M. H., Trimech, M. N., Boussarsar, H., Methamem, M., Marghli, S. & Ltaief, M. Non-invasive pressure support ventilation and CPAP in cardiogenic pulmonary edema: a multicenter randomized study in the emergency department. *Intensive Care Med.* 2011, 37, 249–256.

[14] Ko, D. R., Beom, J., Lee, H. S., You, J. S., Chung, H. S. & Chung, S. P. Benefits of High-Flow Nasal Cannula Therapy for Acute Pulmonary Edema in Patients with Heart Failure in the Emergency Department: A Prospective Multi-Center Randomized Controlled Trial. *J. Clin. Med.* 2020, 9, 1937.

[15] Marjanovic, N., Flacher, A., Drouet, L., Gouhinec, A. Le, Said, H., Vigneau, J.-F., Chollet, B., Lefebvre, S. & Sebbane, M. High-Flow Nasal Cannula in Early Emergency Department Management of Acute Hypercapnic Respiratory Failure Due to Cardiogenic Pulmonary Edema. *Respir. Care* 2020, 65, 1241–1249.

Chapter 14

Respiratory Failure: Non-Invasive Ventilation - Nasal High-Flow Oxygen in Acute Respiratory Distress Syndrome

Mürüvvet Dayıoğlu*, MD
Gazi University Medical Faculty,
Critical Care Fellowship Program, Ankara, Turkey

Abstract

Acute respiratory distress syndrome (ARDS) is a severe feature of acute respiratory failure (ARF) characterized by acute inflammatory lung injury due to increased capillary permeability that is not explained by cardiac causes, defined by Berlin Definition [1, 2]. Besides providing adequate oxygenation, ventilation strategies in order to prevent ventilator-induced lung injury (VILI) and patient self-inflicted lung injury (P-SILI) are an important part of the ventilatory management of ARDS [2].

Like all ARF cases, ARDS may require an escalation therapeutic strategy between conventional oxygen therapy and Extra Corporeal Membrane Oxygenation (ECMO) [2, 3]. Since high-flow nasal cannula (HFNC) and non-invasive ventilation (NIV) are both non-invasive techniques and can be used outside the ICU, they could be good alternatives for patients with mild or moderate ARDS, who are not candidates for invasive mechanical ventilation. Patient selection, and close monitoring via tools like HACOR (Heart rate, Acidosis, Consciousness, Oxygenation, and Respiratory rate) and ROX (Respiratory rate- Oxygenation) could prevent complications [2].

* Corresponding Author's Email: muruvvetd@gmail.com.

In: Nasal High Flow and Non-Invasive Ventilatory Support
Editors: A. M. Esquinas, D. A. Lagonidis, P. Silva Santos et al.
ISBN: 979-8-88697-420-1

Keywords: acute respiratory distress syndrome, ventilator-induced lung injury, patient self-inflicted lung injury, non-invasive ventilation, high-flow nasal cannula

Introduction

Acute respiratory distress syndrome (ARDS), a life-threatening inflammatory lung injury, is defined as acute onset, hypoxia with the partial pressure of arterial oxygen (PaO_2) / fraction off inspiratory oxygen (FiO_2) ratio of less than 300 mmHg, diffuse infiltrates on chest radiography or computed tomography, and respiratory failure not fully explained by the cardiac failure or fluid overload [1].

Maintaining adequate oxygenation remains the mainstay of essential intervention for ARDS. There are potential therapeutic options, including invasive and non-invasive ventilation techniques and ECMO, according to the severity of ARDS purposed [2, 3]. It is also an important strategy to prevent the patient from the complications of ventilators and respiratory drive [2, 3].

It is known that tissue hypoxia, resulting in inflammation, apoptosis and organ dysfunction or failure. Therefore, supportive care for hypoxemia is still crucial for ARDS, however, increased SpO_2 levels was associated with mortality. Therefore, to minimize hyperoa permissive hypoxemia strategy was proposed to minimize hyperoxia-related deleterious effects that lower FiO_2 and target PaO_2 levels associated with long-term cognitive impairment, psychiatric disorders, spite, optimal supplemental oxygen strategy is controversial, $PaO_2 = 65\text{-}75$, $SaO_2 = 90\text{-}95$ is recommended [2].

Since the reduction of respiratory workload and improvement of hypoxemia and therefore, possibility of avoiding endotracheal intubation, NIV and recently HFNC have been area of interest. However, Berlin definition of ARDS include patients who are receiving invasive mechanical ventilation (IMV) and non-invasive mechanical ventilation (NIV) with a tight- fitting mask and positive end expiratory pressure (PEEP) or continuous positive airway pressure (CPAP) of at least 5 cm H_2O, patients who are receiving HFNC do not meet the criterion [1]. Therefore, in ERS/ATS guidelines [4], respiratory failure occurring without prior chronic respiratory disease defined as "de novo ARF" and stated that most patients in this category have hypoxemic respiratory failure, like $PaO_2/FiO_2 \leq 200$ or respiratory rate > 30-35 breath/min. and a non-chronic obstructive pulmonary disease (COPD), like pneumonia and/or ARDS. Because of difficulties due to measurements of actual FiO_2 and PEEP levels, authors preferred to evaluate pneumonia and ARDS in the same group. Recently, Matthay M.A. et al., proposed that the Berlin definition of ARDS be modified to include patients treated with HFNC of at least 30L/ min who meet the other criteria [5].

NIV and HFNC are non-invasive techniques for supporting oxygenation and unloading respiratory muscles. While HFNC provides comfort, NIV is more effective unloading muscles, and they are both effective techniques for mild to moderate ARDS [2]. This chapter focused on oxygen therapy for ARDS, based on an escalation approach.

Non-Invasive Ventilation

Lung protective ventilation which includes low tidal volume, plateau- pressure below 30 cm H_2O, regardless of severity, and PEEP correlated with severity, is recommended for ARDS management [3]. Although the role of NIV in ARDS patients is still controversial, it is used to improve oxygenation, facilitate ventilation, decrease the work of breathing and avoid intubation, and reduce complications associated with invasive mechanical ventilation [2, 4, 6].

Pressure support is necessary to reduce the work of breathing, but especially in patients with high inspiratory demand tidal volume can be exacerbated and can cause P-SILI [2, 4]. A low PEEP causes inefficient oxygenation, but in many studies, PEEP has been used at a 5 mm Hg level, in order to reduce peak pressures or leaks. Therefore, high tidal volume (greater than 9ml/kg) and insufficient pressure support or PEEP settings led to NIV failure [2]. Due to these potential risks and the need for close monitoring, NIV not being recommended for use in these patients, but can be useful in patients who do not increase their tidal volume, despite the uncertainty of evidence [2, 4].

Delayed intubation is the main risk of NIV therapy [2, 7]. The HACOR score is used as an index for predicting NIV failure in ARDS patients. HACOR score >5 was associated with increased hospital mortality [2]. Older age, a higher severity score, presence of moderate-severe ARDS, no improvement after 1 hour of NIV, a decline in PaO_2 / FiO_2 between the first and second day of NIV, and a $PaCO_2$ increase over the first 2 days are found associated with NIV failure [4, 6]. Although careful patient selection, NIV failure is an independent risk factor for mortality in these risk groups. However, patients with PaO_2/ FiO_2 200-300 mm Hg might be successfully managed with NIV [4, 6].

In conclusion, NIV can be a viable alternative for mild and moderate ARDS patients. Patient selection (without shock, multiorgan system failure, abnormal mental status, and severe hypoxia), close monitoring, using scoring tools and experienced clinical team to avoid delayed intubation are important for treatment success [2, 4, 6].

High-Flow Nasal Cannula

HFNC is increasingly popular in place of conventional oxygen therapy for patients with acute hypoxemic respiratory failure. HFNC oxygen rapidly alleviates symptoms of respiratory distress and is considered to have a number of advantages compared with conventional oxygen therapies, including nasopharyngeal CO_2 washout, decreased inspiratory resistance, constant FiO_2, efficient humidification, and PEEP effect [2, 8]. It is known that maintaining adequate oxygenation depends on FiO_2 and PEEP [2, 8]. Conventional devices (nasal cannula and face masks) are flow limited to no more than 15 L/ min, while patients with respiratory failure have high flows between 30 and more than 100L/ min, which results in constant FiO_2. In contrast, HFNC provides more flow, and the difference is reduced and FiO_2 remains relatively constant [8].

Although HFNC is an open system, high flow overcomes resistance against the expiratory flow and HFNC increases nasopharyngeal airway pressure that peaks at the end of expiration and therefore increases airway pressure and therefore lung volume. Airway pressure and lung volume increase proportionally with gas flow. However, mouth opening and closing affect pharyngeal pressure and the PEEP effect remains unclear [2, 8]. In addition, by delivering warm and well-humidified oxygen and by avoiding the discomfort generated NIV masks, HFNC is extremely well tolerated than NIV, which is also a non-invasive technique [2, 8]. Studies suggest that HFNC has fewer adverse effects than NIV and may cause less ventilatory-induced lung injury (VILI) [8].

Clinicians use HFNC to avoid intubation and prevent patients from the harmful effects of IMV. However, studies point out that intubation rates are as high as 30-50% [9] and increasing use of HFNC revealed a risk of delayed intubation, as with NIV [10].

Oxygenation index, known as ROX is a predictive tool for detecting HFNC failure. A ROX index of < 2.85 at 2 h, < 3.47 at 6 h, and < 3.85 at 12 h of initiating HFNC, respectively, were predictors of HFNC failure [11, 12]. HFNC failure is also correlated with Simplified Acute Physiology Score II [12]. Clinical trials demonstrated that HNC can be preferred for mild or moderate hypoxemic ARF, but because it does not guarantee positive pharyngeal pressure, it has not been recommended for severe ARDS [9]. To summarise, HFNC is a good modality for patients with mild to moderate ARDS. Patients must be monitored very closely and when further deterioration or even failure is noticed, should be intubated without delay.

Conclusion

Maintaining adequate oxygenation with lung protective ventilation is essential for the treatment of ARDS patients. Despite controversy, PaO_2 = 65-75, SaO_2 = 90-95 is recommended. NIV and HFNC are both effective techniques for mild to moderate ARDS. Oxygenation, VILI, and P- SILI are the most important cornerstones of ARDS management. Vigilant monitoring is important to avoid delayed intubation, which leads to worse clinical outcomes.

References

[1] ARDS Definition Task Force; V Marco Ranieri, Gordon D Rubenfeld, B Taylor Thompson, Niall D Ferguson, Ellen Caldwell, Eddy Fan, Luigi Camporota, Arthur S Slutsky. 2012. "Acute respiratory distress syndrome: the Berlin Definition." *JAMA*, 307: 2526–33. Accessed 2012 Jun 20. doi:10.1001/jama.2012.5669.

[2] Ohshimo, Shinichiro. 2021. "Oxygen administration for patients with ARDS." *J. Intensive Care*. 9:17. Accessed 2021 Feb 6. doi:10.1186/s40560-021-00532-0.

[3] Niall D Ferguson, Eddy Fan, Luigi Camporota, Massimo Antonelli, Antonio Anzueto, Richard Beale, Laurent Brochard, Roy Brower, Andrés Esteban, Luciano Gattinoni, Andrew Rhodes, Arthur S Slutsky, Jean-Louis Vincent, Gordon D Rubenfeld, B Taylor Thompson, V Marco Ranieri. "The Berlin definition of ARDS: an expanded rationale, justification, and supplementary material Oct;38(10):1731-2]. *Intensive Care Med.* 38:1573-82 Accessed 2012 Agu 25. doi:10.1007/s00134-012-2682-1.

[4] Bram Rochwerg, Laurent Brochard, Mark W Elliott, Dean Hess, Nicholas S Hill, Stefano Nava, Paolo Navalesi Members Of The Steering Committee, Massimo Antonelli, Jan Brozek, Giorgio Conti, Miquel Ferrer, Kalpalatha Guntupalli· Samir Jaber, Sean Keenan, Jordi Mancebo, Sangeeta Mehta, Suhail Raoof Members Of

The Task Force. "Official ERS/ATS clinical practice guidelines: noninvasive ventilation for acute respiratory failure." *Eur. Respir. J.* 50:1602426. Accessed Aug 31, 2017. doi: 10.1183/13993003.02426-2016.

[5] Matthay M A, Thompson B T, Ware L B. 2021. "The Berlin definition of acute respiratory distress syndrome: should patients receiving high-flow nasal oxygen be included?" *Lancet Respir Med.* Aug;9(8):933-936. Accessed Apr 27, 2021. doi: 10.1016/S2213-2600(21)00105-3.

[6] Stephen C Bourke, Thomas Piraino, Lara Pisani, Laurent Brochard, Mark W Elliott. "Beyond the guidelines for non-invasive ventilation in acute respiratory failure: implications for practice." *Lancet Respir. Med.* 6:935-47. Accessed 2018 Dec. doi:10.1016/S2213-2600(18)30388-6.

[7] Alexandre Demoule, Emmanuelle Girou, Jean-Christophe Richard, Solenne Taille, Laurent Brochard .2006. "Benefits and risks of success or failure of noninvasive ventilation." *Intensive Care Med.* Nov;32(11):1756-65. Accessed 2006 Sep 21 doi: 10.1007/s00134-006-0324.

[8] Nishimura, Masaji. 2016. "High-Flow Nasal Cannula Oxygen Therapy in Adults: Physiological Benefits, Indication, Clinical Benefits, and Adverse Effects. "*Respiratory care*, 61: 529–41. Accessed 2016 Apr. doi:10.4187/ respcare. 04577.

[9] Alexandre Demoule, Nicholas Hill, Paolo Navalesi 2016. "Can we prevent intubation in patients with ARDS?" *Intensive Care Med.* May;42(5):768-771. doi: 10.1007/s00134-016-4323-6.

[10] Byung Ju Kang, Younsuck Koh, Chae-Man Lim, Jin Won Huh, Seunghee Baek, Myongja Han, Hyun-Suk Seo, Hee Jung Suh, Ga Jin Seo, Eun Young Kim, Sang-Bum Hong. 2015. "Failure of high-flow nasal cannula therapy may delay intubation and increase mortality." *Intensive Care Med.* Apr;41(4):623-32. Accessed 2015 Feb 18. doi: 10.1007/s00134-015-3693-5.

[11] Oriol Roca, Berta Caralt, Jonathan Messika, Manuel Samper, Benjamin Sztrymf, Gonzalo Hernández, Marina García-de-Acilu, Jean-Pierre Frat, Joan R Masclans, Jean-Damien Ricard. 2019. "An index combining respiratory rateand oxygenation to predict outcome of nasal high-flow therapy." *Am. J. Respir. Crit. Care Med.* 199(11):1368–76. June 1.doi: 10.1164/rccm.201803-0589OC.

[12] Jonathan Messika, Karim Ben Ahmed, Stéphane Gaudry, Romain Miguel-Montanes, Cédric Rafat, Benjamin Sztrymf, Didier Dreyfuss, Jean-Damien Ricard, 2015 "Use of High-Flow Nasal Cannula Oxygen Therapy in Subjects With ARDS: A 1-Year Observational Study." *Respir. Care.* 60:162-9. Accessed 2014 Nov 4. doi: 10.4187/respcare.03423.

Chapter 15

Acute Hypoxemic Respiratory Failure: Interstitial Lung Disease

Filipa Jesus*, MD
Pulmonology Department,
Local Health Unit of the E.P.E., Guarda, Portugal

Abstract

Interstitial lung diseases (ILDs) are a broad and heterogeneous group of diseases, whose natural history is characterized by an insidious progression to chronic respiratory failure (CRF) or by life-threatening episodes of acute respiratory failure (ARF). During ARF there is a high degree of diffusion impairment, with hypoxemia and a need for oxygen supplementation. When this is not enough, High-Flow Nasal Cannula (HFNC), Non-invasive Ventilation (NIV) or Invasive Mechanical Ventilation (IMV) arise as treatments that can be used.

Current guidelines recommend that most patients with respiratory failure should not receive IMV due to the negative clinical outcomes. On the other hand, the use of NIV in ARF in selected patients that responded favorably to this therapy was associated with better outcomes and survival rates. When HFNC was compared with NIV no differences were found in the intubation rate and mortality.

Chronic respiratory failure (CRF) is often part of the clinical course of ILDs, and as the disease progresses there is a growing impairment in gas exchange, leading to respiratory failure with hypoxemia. In this situation, the use of NIV and HFNC might also present various applications, from palliation to bridge to lung transplant. Future studies are needed to elucidate its best application.

* Corresponding Author's Email: filipa.jesus@ulsguarda.min-saude.pt.

In: Nasal High Flow and Non-Invasive Ventilatory Support
Editors: A. M. Esquinas, D. A. Lagonidis, P. Silva Santos et al.
ISBN: 979-8-88697-420-1

Keywords: idiopathic pulmonary fibrosis, acute respiratory failure, chronic respiratory failure, high-flow nasal cannula, non-invasive ventilation

Introduction

Interstitial lung diseases (ILDs) are a broad and heterogeneous group of diseases characterized by fibrotic and/or inflammatory abnormalities of the lung parenchyma. These conditions share the propensity to cause breathlessness and/or cough and are associated with bilateral abnormal opacities seen in chest radiographs or chest computed tomography [1].

The typical patient presents with a history of progressively worsening exertional dyspnea and persistent non-productive cough, evolving in a slower or faster way to respiratory failure. Hence, the natural history of ILDs can be characterized by an insidious progression to chronic respiratory failure or by life-threatening episodes of acute respiratory failure [2].

ILDs can be classified based on their onset (acute vs chronic), severity (mild to severe) and reversibility (reversible or irreversible). Besides this, they can also be divided into ILDs with known etiology, such as connective tissue diseases, drugs or other environmental exposures, or unknown etiology (idiopathic interstitial pneumonias, sarcoidosis, and others).

As the classification of ILDs has been revised, epidemiological data is not very precise. A large study estimated that the prevalence of ILD in men was 81/100000 and in females was 64/100000. It also showed a higher incidence in males (31,5/100000 per year) than in females (26,1/100000 per year) [3]. The most common ILDs are idiopathic pulmonary fibrosis (IPF) and sarcoidosis, and, therefore, are the ones more studied.

Regarding the prognosis of ILDs, IPF has the worst prognosis, with a mean survival of 2 to 3 years after the diagnosis and nearly all patients have died within 6 years of diagnosis, mainly due to acute exacerbations of IPF [4]. Connective tissue disease related ILD has a better prognosis than IPF and sarcoidosis is the ILDs with the best prognosis [5].

Acute Respiratory Failure

Acute respiratory failure (ARF) can be the form of presentation of an ILD, although this is less common. It can represent the onset of a new rapidly progressive ILD, namely acute interstitial pneumonia, cryptogenic organizing pneumonia, acute eosinophilic pneumonia or diffuse alveolar hemorrhage, or the clinical onset of an underdiagnosed ILD, in which previous signs and symptoms have gone unnoticed [5].

The rapid decline in respiratory function that characterizes the ARF may occur as a result of an accelerated worsening of the underlying interstitial process – acute exacerbation (AE) – or as a result of a superimposed complication or decompensation of a comorbidity.

The most studied acute exacerbation of an underlying ILD is the acute exacerbation of IPF (AE-IPF), and it has been defined as an acute (< 1 month) respiratory deterioration in a previously diagnosed IPF patient, with exclusion of alternative etiologies (such as infection, heart failure or pulmonary embolism) [6]. The incidence of AE-IPF goes up to 21% and occurs mainly in advanced stages of the disease. Risk factors for AE-IPF are lower forced vital capacity, lower diffusion capacity of carbon monoxide (DLCO) and reduced walked distance at 6-min walking test. The in-hospital mortality rate of an AE-IPF is around 50%, and afterwards mean survival ranges go up to 4 months [6]. During ARF there is a high degree of diffusion impairment and a V/Q mismatch, hence, to avoid hypoxemia, high levels of oxygen are needed. Therefore, the basis of treatment is oxygen supplementation, that, depending on the degree of respiratory failure, can be delivered in different forms and quantities. It goes from simple nasal cannulae to face masks, namely Ventury masks and high concentration oxygen with reservoir mask [5].

Usually, in respiratory failure of ILDs there is an increase in the respiratory rate as a compensatory mechanism, and consequently, the risk of hypercapnia is very little and only on late disease stages [7]. When the abovementioned options are not enough, High Flow Nasal Cannula (HFNC), Non-invasive Ventilation (NIV) or Invasive Mechanical Ventilation (IMV) arise as treatments that can be used. Compared to conventional supplementation with oxygen, HFNC can provide high flows of oxygen, with up to 100% of FiO2 delivered. Besides this, it has a carbon dioxide washout effect and reduces dead space, leading to a reduced ventilatory drive, decreased respiratory rate and work of breathing [8]. Other benefits described with the use of HFNC are positive airway pressure effect, secretion clearance and reduction in intubation rate [8].

The ARF can be so severe that patients might need intensive care support, specifically IMV. The beneficial effects of IMV, namely the recruitment of poorly ventilated alveoli, unload of respiratory muscles and favorable hemodynamic impact on coexisting acute heart failure, might seem enough reasons to utilize this ventilatory support. However, studies have shown that the use of IMV is associated with negative clinical outcomes, reaching an in-hospital mortality higher than 90% [9]. In fact, current IPF guidelines recommend that the majority of patients with respiratory failure should not receive IMV [4]. This is based on the fact that the forces applied through IMV lead to pathophysiological alterations culminating in the disruption of cell membranes and cell-cell contacts, explaining the high susceptibility of these patients to ventilator-induced lung injury (VILI) and, subsequently, the high mortality rate of ILD patients in the ICU [5].

Despite the majority of studies having been conducted on AE-IPF, studies show that AEs of non-IPF forms of ILD do not differ in terms of prognosis [10].

Non-invasive ventilation emerges as a feasible alternative to IMV and may be applied to these patients with the objective of trying to treat or stabilize the cause of ARF and as a mean to avoid intubation, minimizing the risk of its and IMV complications (namely ventilation-induced pneumonia) [5]. On the same way that ILDs are a heterogeneous group of diseases, the response to NIV differs from patient to patient.

Numerous studies have been made in order to evaluate the use of NIV in ARF, showing that in the patients that responded favorably, the use of NIV was associated with better outcomes and survival rates. This responsiveness was associated with less severe ARF and early NIV initiation during the acute phase, indicating that early optimization may improve patients' outcomes. On the other hand, in those that NIV failed, the prognostic was poor, with survival rates of less than 3 months. Failure was more common in patients that needed continuous NIV and did not tolerate interruptions for feeding [11].

Alberti et al., tried to evaluate the response to NIV in ILDs according to ARF etiology and to the underlying radiological pattern of ILD. They showed that when the cause of the ARF is a potentially reversible trigger, for example pneumonia, NIV improved oxygenation, nevertheless this was not translated into a better clinical outcome. When the cause of ARF was AE, NIV could not have any positive impact. Besides this, when they analyzed the response to NIV in terms of radiological pattern, no differences were observed [2]. This study suggests that in clinical practice, the use of NIV in ARF of an ILD should be individualized. A trial of NIV could be considered in patients where the cause is pneumonia, although no favorable impact on clinical outcomes has been proven [2]. More studies are needed in this area, with larger populations and in a controlled setting, to confirm this information.

However, although some studies have been able to show the effectiveness of NIV treating ARF in ILDs, in most of these patients, the excessive work of breathing cannot be managed by NIV alone, and studies suggesting a definitive clinical benefit of NIV in ILDs are still lacking [5].

In patients in which respiratory insufficiency persists despite the use of NIV, there is hemodynamic instability, the patient has severely altered consciousness, or presents with an immediate need for endotracheal intubation, IMV must be considered. When HFNC was compared with NIV no differences were found in the rate of intubation and mortality [5].

In terms of ventilatory modes and settings in NIV, the usual ventilatory mode used is pressure support ventilation, though there are not many studies approaching this issue.

As mentioned before, ARF in these patients is characterized by deep hypoxemia in the first stage and carbon dioxide retention due to respiratory fatigue in the second stage. Therefore, usually Continuous Positive Airway Pressure (CPAP) or HFNC may be applied in the first stage, when patients present with severe acute respiratory failure (PaO_2/FiO_2 ratio less than 250) and signs of respiratory distress, in the absence of respiratory acidosis ($pH < 7.35$, $PaCO_2 \geq 45$ mmHg) [5].

When the patient shows signs of respiratory fatigue (second stage), with respiratory acidosis ($pH < 7.35$, $PaCO_2 \geq 45$ mmHg), or has other conditions that predispose to respiratory insufficiency with hypercapnia (for example, COPD), bi-level NIV is used [5].

There are several difficulties that we can encounter with NIV in ILDs patients. One of the most frequent ones is the fact that many of these patients have fibrotic lungs, with an increased risk of pneumothorax, and so, we need to be cautious with the high pressures during ventilation. On the other hand, it is difficult to obtain adequate tidal volumes due to these fibrotic lungs, so we need to find a balance in order to obtain acceptable minute ventilation, in which we have low tidal volumes but increased respiratory rate. In addition to this, in order to avoid further damage and overdistension of the lung, we need to set low to moderate positive end-expiratory pressures (PEEP) [5].

In relation with this, another problem that arises frequently in ILDs patients requiring non-invasive ventilation is their high respiratory rate, which generates patient-ventilator asynchrony, leading to inefficacy of ventilation with negative clinical outcomes. This increased respiratory rate is a means to achieve adequate minute ventilation, as mentioned before, but can also result of the intense breathlessness reported by the patients, especially in the acute phase. Strategies to solve this problem are the use of drugs to control the respiratory rate, namely opiates (with caution, to avoid over-depressing the respiratory center), set a rapid inspiratory curve in the ventilator or increase the fraction of inspired oxygen (FiO_2) [5].

In conclusion, despite the high rate of NIV failure in patients with ILDs and ARF, in selected patients, such as those with less severe respiratory failure, an early NIV trial might facilitate the recognition of NIV-responder patients, who may benefit from its use. That being said, it is important to remember that ILD patients represent a population that suffers from high morbidity and mortality, and where therapeutic options are very limited especially in the presence of ARF. These patients suffer multiple times from intense dyspnea, that doesn't resolve with simple supplementary oxygen. Therefore, NIV also emerges as a palliative measure to relieve dyspnea, as explained in more detail below.

Chronic Respiratory Failure

Chronic respiratory failure (CRF) is often part of the clinical course of ILDs, as a result of the worsening of the underlying disease or caused by decompensation of its associated comorbidities [7].

As the ILD progresses, there is a progressive impairment in gas exchange, due to the decrease in diffusion capacity and alteration in the ventilation-perfusion ratio, resulting in an increased alveolar-arterial oxygen gradient. This reflects functionally, with a decrease in diffusion capacity for carbon dioxide. Chronically, this leads to respiratory failure with hypoxemia, resulting in an increase in respiratory rate as a compensatory mechanism, with hypercapnia developing only in the late disease stages. Besides this, as the disease progresses, there is an extracellular matrix deposition, with an increase in lung elastic recoil and consequently an increase in the respiratory rate. This initially minimizes the work of breathing, however in the late stages, with a slight increase in exercise intensity there is an increase in physiological dead space, leading to a bigger respiratory request and possible hypercapnia [7].

Another mechanism contributing to CRF is pulmonary vascular damage. The reason for this damage is the sharp increase in pulmonary pressures that happens during exercise due to the hypoxic pulmonary vasoconstriction. With disease progression, this vascular damage increases, leading to a reduction in vascular bed, an increase of right ventricular afterload and, eventually, heart failure with early oxyhemoglobin desaturation [7].

As mentioned before, the natural history of ILDs can be characterized by insidious progression to CRF or, more rarely, by life-threatening episodes of ARF [2]. The time between the diagnosis of the ILD and the development of CRF is variable, depending on the velocity of disease progression. For example, IPF is characterized by a more rapid progression, with an early onset of respiratory failure, while some Connective tissue disease-associated interstitial lung diseases (CTD-ILD) progress slowly, with the patient never developing CRF. Not rarely, patients get used to hypoxemia and adjust their daily life, thus, chronic respiratory failure and disease progression needs to be investigated every consultation. This investigation is made with arterial blood gases analysis, pulmonary function tests, six-minute walking test (6MWT) and high resolution computed tomography (HRCT). Disease progression can be defined by a decline in forced vital capacity of $\geq 10\%$ or in DLCO of $\geq 15\%$ over 6 months or by an increase in disease extent in HRCT [12].

Chronic respiratory failure can also be associated with the decompensation of comorbidities or development of complications related with ILDs. In this case, the management of CRF involves optimizing and treating these comorbidities.

One of these complications is pulmonary hypertension (PH), defined as mean pulmonary artery pressure ≥ 25 mmHg and confirmed by right heart catheterization (RHC). Despite RHC being the gold standard for the diagnosis of PH, echocardiography is used more commonly as a screening tool, due to its accessibility and the fact that is non-invasive. PH is common in IPF, with a prevalence up to 86%, and should be suspected when the patient has resting, or exertional dyspnea and hypoxemia not fully explained by the degree of impairment of lung parenchyma [13]. Currently, there are no approved therapies for the treatment of PH in IPF patients, thus, the treatment consists of supportive measures, such as supplementary oxygen to correct hypoxemia, diuretics, and treatment of contributing factors, such as obstructive sleep apnea syndrome (OSAS).

Other complications that should be monitored and treated include pulmonary embolism, COPD, small airways disease, OSAS and congestive heart failure.

Patients with ILDs have an increased risk of pulmonary embolism (PE) due to their pro-coagulant and inflammatory state and their prolonged immobility, secondary to exertional dyspnea and joint or muscle pain (in CTD-ILD) [7]. Cardiovascular diseases and congestive heart failure also represent a common comorbidity in ILDs patients, as these pathologies multiple times share the same risk factors (advanced age and smoking exposure, in IPF patients). These comorbidities should be suspected when the patient refers to dyspnea disproportionate to the severity and extent of underlying ILD and refers other symptoms, for example chest pain or angina [7].

After optimization and treatment of these comorbidities, if chronic respiratory failure maintains it may be necessary to initiate oxygen supplementation. Despite not having evidence in improving survival, oxygen therapy is recommended for hypoxemic patients in guidelines [4]. It has been shown to improve exercise tolerance, symptoms, and quality of life [14]. When simple oxygen supplementation is not enough to correct the patient's hypoxemia, similarly to ARF, HFNC can be an option, with the same beneficial physiological effects as mentioned above (carbon dioxide washout, PEEP effect and secretion clearance) [8].

Non-invasive ventilation is another option when supplemental oxygen is insufficient. In the same way as with oxygen and HFNC, NIV cannot modify the natural history of ILDs, but improves symptoms, namely dyspnea, and quality of life. Besides this, it has a significant role in end-stage ILD, when hypercapnic chronic respiratory failure might be established. In these situations, chronic use of nocturnal bi-level NIV can decrease daytime arterial pressure of carbon dioxide and increase arterial partial pressure of oxygen [15].

Furthermore, HFNC and NIV can have a role regarding palliative care in ILDs, helping to control dyspnea. This is one of the most common symptoms in the advanced stages of ILDs, and given the abovementioned advantages of these therapies, they might have a role in the management of CRF for patients with severe hypoxemia [7]. Alongside these ventilatory supports, opioids and benzodiazepines are also used, what may seem incongruous, however it aims to reduce respiratory rate, optimize patient-ventilator adaptation, and with this, reducing refractory dyspnea.

When HFNC was compared with NIV, HFNC was associated with an equivalent survival rate, better tolerance, less temporary interruption, and discontinuation rates, allowing patients to eat and talk. This suggests that HFNC might be a good choice in palliative treatment in ILD patients [7].

NIV was also used as a ventilatory support to patients with ILD during rehabilitation, with satisfactory results, increasing exercise tolerability and decreasing dyspnea and cardiac effort [7]. However, more studies are needed in order to evaluate this possible use of NIV.

Independently of the specific ILD, lung transplantation is currently the only effective treatment to patients with advanced ILD, whilst oxygen supplementation and ventilatory support are only supportive measures. A timely referral to transplant center is very important, because the wait can be long and not on time, due to the reduced number of available organs. Moreover, there are several exams that need to be done previous to the transplant and the patient needs to gain strong psychosocial support. In patients with advanced ILD with CRF, while they wait for a compatible organ, NIV and HFNC can be used as a bridge to transplant, allowing the patient to survive. However, this is not feasible during a long period of time since the disease progresses and there are limits to where these supportive measures can sustain the patient [7].

In summary, the use of NIV and HFNC in CRF in ILD patients might present very different fields of application, from palliation or bridge to transplant to rehabilitation programs. Nevertheless, given the paucity of studies and the low quality of the evidence available, future studies are needed to elucidate its best application.

Conclusion

Interstitial lung diseases (ILDs) are a broad and heterogeneous group of diseases with a propensity to cause breathlessness and/or cough. Due to diffusion impairment, the natural history of ILDs can be characterized by an insidious progression to chronic respiratory failure or by life-threatening episodes of acute respiratory failure. During acute respiratory failure there is a high degree of diffusion impairment, with hypoxemia and a need for oxygen supplementation. When this is not enough, High Flow Nasal Cannula (HFNC), Non-invasive Ventilation (NIV) or Invasive Mechanical Ventilation (IMV) arise as treatments that can be used.

Current guidelines recommend that the majority of patients with respiratory failure should not receive IMV due to the negative clinical outcomes. On the other hand, the use of NIV in ARF in selected patients that responded favorably to an early NIV trial was associated with better outcomes and survival rates. When HFNC was compared with NIV no differences were found in the intubation rate and mortality.

There are several difficulties that we can encounter with NIV in ILDs patients, namely an increased risk of pneumothorax, difficulty to obtain adequate tidal volumes and a high respiratory rate, generating patient-ventilator asynchrony. There are several strategies that can be adopted, such as the adjustment of ventilator settings and the use of drugs. Chronic respiratory failure (CRF) is often part of the clinical course of ILDs, and as the disease progresses there is a growing impairment in gas exchange, leading to respiratory failure with hypoxemia. In this situation, the use of NIV and HFNC might also present various applications, from palliation to bridge to lung transplant. Future studies are needed to elucidate its best application.

References

[1] Travis W D, Costabel U, Hansell D M, King T E Jr, Lynch D A, Nicholson A G, Ryerson C J, Ryu J H, Selman M, Wells A U, Behr J, Bouros D, Brown K K, Colby T V, Collard H R, Cordeiro C R, Cottin V, Crestani B, Drent M, Dudden RF, Egan J, Flaherty K, Hogaboam C, Inoue Y, Johkoh T, Kim D S, Kitaichi M, Loyd J, Martinez F J, Myers J, Protzko S, Raghu G, Richeldi L, Sverzellati N, Swigris J, Valeyre D; ATS/ERS Committee on Idiopathic Interstitial Pneumonias. An official American Thoracic Society/European Respiratory Society statement: Update of the international multidisciplinary classification of the idiopathic interstitial pneumonias. *Am. J. Respir. Crit. Care Med.* 2013 Sep 15;188(6):733-48. doi: 10. 1164/rccm.201308-1483ST.

[2] Aliberti S, Messinesi G, Gamberini S, Maggiolini S, Visca D, Galavotti V, Giuliani F, Cosentini R, Brambilla AM, Blasi F, Scala R, Carone M, Luisi F, Harari S, Voza A, Esquinas A, Pesci A. Non-invasive mechanical ventilation in patients with diffuse interstitial lung diseases. *BMC Pulm. Med.* 2014 Dec 5;14:194. doi: 10.1186/1471-2466-14-194.

[3] Coultas DB, Zumwalt RE, Black WC, Sobonya RE. The epidemiology of interstitial lung diseases. *Am. J. Respir. Crit. Care Med.* 1994 Oct;150(4):967-72. doi: 10.1164/ajrccm.150.4.7921471.

[4] Raghu G, Rochwerg B, Zhang Y, Garcia CA, Azuma A, Behr J, Brozek J L, Collard HR, Cunningham W, Homma S, Johkoh T, Martinez F J, Myers J, Protzko S L, Richeldi L, Rind D, Selman M, Theodore A, Wells AU, Hoogsteden H, Schünemann HJ; American Thoracic Society; European Respiratory society; Japanese Respiratory Society; Latin American Thoracic Association. An Official ATS/ERS/JRS/ALAT Clinical Practice Guideline: Treatment of Idiopathic Pulmonary Fibrosis. An Update of the 2011 Clinical Practice Guideline. *Am. J. Respir. Crit. Care Med.* 2015 Jul 15;192(2):e3-19. doi: 10.1164/rccm.201506-1063ST. Erratum in: *Am. J. Respir. Crit. Care Med.* 2015 Sep 1;192(5):644. Dosage error in article text.

[5] Faverio P, De Giacomi F, Sardella L, Fiorentino G, Carone M, Salerno F, Ora J, Rogliani P, Pellegrino G, Sferrazza Papa GF, Bini F, Bodini BD, Messinesi G, Pesci A, Esquinas A. Management of acute respiratory failure in interstitial lung diseases: overview and clinical insights. *BMC Pulm. Med.* 2018 May 15;18(1):70. doi: 10.1186/s12890-018-0643-3.

[6] Collard H R, Ryerson C J, Corte T J, Jenkins G, Kondoh Y, Lederer D J, Lee J S, Maher TM, Wells AU, Antoniou K M, Behr J, Brown K K, Cottin V, Flaherty K R, Fukuoka J, Hansell D M, Johkoh T, Kaminski N, Kim DS, Kolb M, Lynch DA,

Myers JL, Raghu G, Richeldi L, Taniguchi H, Martinez FJ. Acute Exacerbation of Idiopathic Pulmonary Fibrosis. An International Working Group Report. *Am. J. Respir. Crit. Care Med.* 2016 Aug 1;194(3):265-75. doi: 10.1164/rccm.201604-0801CI.

[7] Faverio P, De Giacomi F, Bonaiti G, Stainer A, Sardella L, Pellegrino G, Sferrazza Papa G F, Bini F, Bodini B D, Carone M, Annoni S, Messinesi G, Pesci A. Management of Chronic Respiratory Failure in Interstitial Lung Diseases: Overview and Clinical Insights. *Int. J. Med. Sci.* 2019 Jun 10;16(7):967-980. doi: 10.7150/ijms.32752.

[8] Bräunlich J, Beyer D, Mai D, Hammerschmidt S, Seyfarth H J, Wirtz H. Effects of nasal high flow on ventilation in volunteers, COPD and idiopathic pulmonary fibrosis patients. *Respiration*. 2013;85(4):319-25. doi: 10.1159/000342027. *Epub* 2012 Nov 1.

[9] Al-Hameed, Sharma S. Outcome of patients admitted to the intensive care unit for acute exacerbation of idiopathic pulmonary fibrosis. *Can. Respir. J.* 2004 Mar;11(2):117-22. doi: 10.1155/2004/379723.

[10] Fernández-Pérez E R, Yilmaz M, Jenad H, Daniels C E, Ryu J H, Hubmayr R D, Gajic O. Ventilator settings and outcome of respiratory failure in chronic interstitial lung disease. *Chest.* 2008 May;133(5):1113-9. doi: 10.1378/chest.07-1481. *Epub* 2007 Nov 7.

[11] Yokoyama T, Tsushima K, Yamamoto H, Koizumi T, Kubo K. Potential benefits of early continuous positive pressure ventilation in patients with rapidly progressive interstitial pneumonia. *Respirology.* 2012 Feb;17(2):315-21. doi: 10.1111/j.1440-1843.2011.02051.x.

[12] Robbie H, Daccord C, Chua F, Devaraj A. Evaluating disease severity in idiopathic pulmonary fibrosis. *Eur. Respir. Rev.* 2017 Sep 6;26(145):170051. doi: 10.1183/16000617.0051-2017.

[13] Raghu G, Amatto V C, Behr J, Stowasser S. Comorbidities in idiopathic pulmonary fibrosis patients: a systematic literature review. *Eur. Respir. J.* 2015 Oct;46(4):1113-30. doi: 10.1183/13993003.02316-2014.

[14] Egan J J. Follow-up and nonpharmacological management of the idiopathic pulmonary fibrosis patient. *Eur. Respir. Rev.* 2011 Jun;20(120):114-7. doi: 10.1183/09059180.00001811.

[15] Koschel D, Handzhiev S, Wiedemann B, Höffken G. Acute effects of NPPV in interstitial lung disease with chronic hypercapnic respiratory failure. *Respir Med.* 2010 Feb;104(2):291-5. doi: 10.1016/j.rmed.2009.09.017. *Epub* 2009 Oct 17.

Chapter 16

Mechanical Stretch and Ventilator-Induced Lung Injury Pathophysiology and Clinical Implications in Non-Invasive Ventilation

Marta Duarte-Silva[1,*], MD
João Rodrigues[1], MD
Dionisio Maia[1], MD
and António Miguel[1], MD
[1] Hospital de Santa Marta,
Hospital and University Center of Central Lisbon, Lisbon, Portugal

Abstract

Despite the clear benefits of non-invasive ventilation in acute and chronic respiratory failure, the lung can be injured by being stretched excessively. The major injuries associated with physical force that cause ventilator-induced lung injury (VILI) are "volutrauma" and "atelectotrauma." Imposed loads from inappropriate NIV settings can also affect the respiratory center and lead to trigger and cycling asynchronies.

It is important to understand these concepts to use strategies that minimize ventilator-induced lung injury and reduce subsequent development of pulmonary fibrosis.

Keywords: mechanical stretch, mechanoreceptors, non-invasive ventilation, asynchrony, ventilator-induced lung injury

---

[*] Corresponding Author's Email: maria.silva42@chlc.min-saude.pt.

In: Nasal High Flow and Non-Invasive Ventilatory Support
Editors: A. M. Esquinas, D. A. Lagonidis, P. Silva Santos et al.
ISBN: 979-8-88697-420-1

Effects of Non-Invasive Ventilation on Muscle Loading and the Respiratory Center

To understand the pathophysiology of mechanical stretch in the lung, it is important to review the anatomical and functional mechanisms underlying the regulation of breathing.

The ventilatory pattern (tidal volume, frequency, and inspiratory/ expiratory ratio) is controlled by the respiratory center located in the brain stem. The respiratory center has an inherent respiratory rhythm generator that interacts with several inputs [2]. Two important inputs come from chemoreceptors (not reviewed in this chapter) and from mechanoreceptors, located in the muscular portions of the walls of the bronchi and bronchioles.

These are stretch receptors that transmit signals through the vagus nerve into the dorsal respiratory group of neurons when the lungs become over-stretched. These signals limit inspiration, that is, when the lungs become excessively inflated, the stretch receptors activate an appropriate feedback response that "switches off" the inspiratory ramp and thus stops further inspiration.

This mechanism is called the Hering-Breuer inflation reflex [1]. This reflex increases the rate of respiration as it shortens expiration and the entire period of each respiratory cycle. In humans the Hering-Bruer reflex is not activated until the tidal volume increases to more than 3x normal (>1.5L/breath). It is a protective mechanism for preventing excess lung inflation [1].

The purpose of mechanical ventilation is to rest the respiratory muscles and provide an adequate gas exchange. This patient-ventilator interaction has profound effects on the patient´s respiratory centre. Muscle unloading will often reduce the intensity and timing of the mechanical inputs sensed by the respiratory centre, decreasing minute ventilation and work of breathing. Nocturnal unloading of chronically overloaded muscles may reset the respiratory centre targets for a more normal $PaCO_2$ and VA during the day.

Imposed loads from inappropriate NIV settings can therefore affect the respiratory centre and lead to trigger and cycling asynchronies. If overventilation and overdistention are sensed through mechanoreceptors during flow delivery, this will lead to shortening of neural inspiratory time and even activation of expiratory muscles during the inspiratory fase, resulting in increased dyspnea. Additionally, delayed or missed triggers are sensed as an uncomfortable isometric load leading to increased effort intensity [2].

Mechanical Stretch and Ventilator-Induced Lung Injury

Every time a person takes a breath, the pressure necessary to inflate the lung comprises the pressure to overcome airway resistance, and the pressure to overcome the elastic properties of the lung. At end-inspiration, when airflow is zero, the main force maintaining inflation is the transpulmonary pressure (alveolar pressure minus pleural pressure) [3]. Thus, lung volume and transpulmonary pressure are inextricably linked. When a musician plays the trumpet, airway pressure can reach 150 cm of water [4], but pneumothorax is uncommon because pleural pressure is also elevated, hence there is no increase in transpulmonary pressure. On the other hand, during non-invasive ventilation, if the patient is in distress and generating a large negative pleural pressure, transpulmonary pressure may be extremely with accompanying lung overdistension [3].

Despite the clear benefits of non-invasive ventilation in acute and chronic respiratory insufficiency, the lung can be injured because of being stretched excessively. The major injuries associated with a physical force that cause ventilator-induced lung injury (VILI) are "volutrauma" and "atelectotrauma."

When ventilation occurs with high lung volumes, alveolar overdistension can lead to increased alveolar-capillary permeability with pulmonary oedema, alveolar rupture, air leaks and gross barotrauma (e.g., pneumothorax, pneumomediastinum, and subcutaneous emphysema). Dreyfuss *et al.* [5]. found that pulmonary oedema developed in animals undergoing ventilation with high tidal volumes, whereas such oedema did not occur in animals undergoing ventilation with similar airway pressures but with straps around their abdomen and chests that reduced tidal volumes. Thus, their experiments showed that volume (i.e., lung stretching), not airway pressure, was the most crucial factor in determining injury.

When ventilation occurs at low lung volumes, lung injury can be caused by the repetitive opening and closing of the airways and lung units, effects of surfactant function, and regional hypoxia. This type of injury, "atelectotrauma," is characterized by epithelial sloughing, hyaline membranes, and pulmonary oedema [3]. Mead et al. observed that the stretching forces in lung parenchyma at margins between aerated and atelectatic regions could be up to 4-5x as high as those in other lung regions [6].

These forms of ventilator-induced lung injury manifest pathologically as diffuse alveolar damage and are associated with cytokine release and bacterial translocation. Furthermore, experimental advances have significantly increased the understanding of the process of mechanotransduction in lung cells. In vitro studies have shown that the mechanical forces induce extracellular matrix expression with increasing procollagen fiber expression [9]. Thus, protective ventilatory strategies are essential to reduce any early stimulus for fibrogenesis.

Interactions of respiratory system mechanics and mechanical ventilation strategies to minimize lung injury include low tidal volumes to limit overdistention and higher PEEPs to prevent injury from low lung volume. In the ARDS Network study (2000) [7], ventilation with a lower tidal volume (6ml per kilogram of predicted body weight) and limited plateau pressure to 30cm of water showed a decreased mortality and increased the number of days without ventilator use. A 2012 meta-analysis showed that among patients without ARDS, protective ventilation with lower tidal volumes was also associated with better clinical outcomes [8].

A clinical challenge with NIV occurs when ventilator settings are minimal, yet a vigorous patient effort results in potentially harmful transpulmonary pressures and volumes. Under these circumstances, reversible causes of this inspiratory effort (e.g., pain, acidosis, anxiety) must be addressed. Beyond that, however, management of such patients without obvious causes is problematic.

Conclusion

Imposed loads from inappropriate NIV settings can affect the respiratory centre and lead to trigger and cycling asynchronies. Alveolar overdistension can lead to increased alveolar-capillary permeability with pulmonary oedema, alveolar rupture, air leaks and gross barotrauma. Stretching forces in lung parenchyma at margins between aerated and atelectatic regions are much higher than those in other lung regions. Lung-protective strategies should be adopted in all patients, however, the ideal ventilation strategy remains to be determined.

References

[1] Hall JE. (2015). *Guyton and Hall Textbook of Medical Physiology*. Elsevier Gezondheidszorg.

[2] MacIntyre NR. (2019, May 20). Physiologic Effects of Noninvasive Ventilation. *Respiratory Care,* 64(6), 617-628. https://doi.org/10.4187/respcare.06635.

[3] Slutsky AS and Ranieri VM. (2013, November 28). Ventilator-Induced Lung Injury. *New England Journal of Medicine*, 369(22), 2126-2136. https://doi.org/10.1056/nejmra1208707.

[4] Bouhuys A. (1969, March). Physiology and Musical Instruments. *Nature,* 221(5187), 1199-1204. https://doi.org/10.1038/2211199a0.

[5] Dreyfuss D, Soler P, Basset G and Saumon G. (1988, May). High Inflation Pressure Pulmonary Edema: Respective Effects of High Airway Pressure, High Tidal Volume, and Positive End-expiratory Pressure. *American Review of Respiratory Disease,* 137(5), 1159-1164. https://doi.org/10.1164/ajrccm/137.5.1159.

[6] Mead J, Takishima T and Leith D. (1970, May). Stress distribution in lungs: A model of pulmonary elasticity. *Journal of Applied Physiology*, 28(5), 596-608. https://doi.org/10.1152/jappl.1970.28.5.596.

[7] Ventilation with Lower Tidal Volumes as Compared with Traditional Tidal Volumes for Acute Lung Injury and the Acute Respiratory Distress Syndrome. (2000, May 4). *New England Journal of Medicine*, 342(18), 1301-1308. https://doi.org/10.1056/nejm200005043421801.

[8] Serpa Neto A, Cardoso SO, Manetta JA, Pereira VGM, Espósito DC, Pasqualucci MDOP, Damasceno MCT and Schultz MJ. (2012, October 24). Association Between Use of Lung-Protective Ventilation with Lower Tidal Volumes and Clinical Outcomes among Patients without Acute Respiratory Distress Syndrome. *JAMA,* 308(16), 1651. https://doi.org/10.1001/jama.2012.13730.

[9] Garcia C, Prota L, Morales M, Romero P, Zin W and Rocco P. (2006, June). Understanding the mechanisms of lung mechanical stress. *Brazilian Journal of Medical and Biological Research,* 39(6), 697-706. https://doi.org/10.1590/s0100-879x2006000600001.

Chapter 17

Do-Not-Intubate in Cancer: Hematologic Malignancy Patients

Yerosimou Fotis[*], MD
Charatsis Christos, MD
and Eirini Papageorgiou, MD
Intensive Care Unit, "Theagenio" Cancer Hospital, Thessaloniki, Greece

Abstract

Cancer management and treatment procedures are constantly advancing with newer chemotherapeutic agents, evolved surgical techniques as well as more targeted treatments. It is estimated that 40% of patients will suffer from respiratory failure. There is only a small percentage of patients with directives and decisions concerning a Do-Not-Intubate (DNI) order. Refusing intubation is not the same as refusing resuscitation and the patients must be kept informed about their options.

Intubation and admission in the Intensive Care Unit (ICU) could be beneficial for some patients. While intubation and invasive mechanical ventilation is a cornerstone of supportive treatment for acute respiratory failure, a proportion of patients do not receive invasive mechanical ventilation. There has been evolvement in the patient selection that will benefit from admission in the ICU. Many patients with end-stage cancer that do not want futile treatment and procedures towards their end of life can sign legal orders such as "do-not-intubate" or "do-not-resuscitate" (DNR). When simple oxygen mask will not suffice, the physician must support the patient with alternative ways to provide maximal comfort and as little stress as possible.

---

[*] Corresponding Author's Email: yerosimoufotis@yahoo.com.

In: Nasal High Flow and Non-Invasive Ventilatory Support
Editors: A. M. Esquinas, D. A. Lagonidis, P. Silva Santos et al.
ISBN: 979-8-88697-420-1

In cases of a DNI order, the physician may use non-invasive ventilation (NIV) and high-flow nasal cannula (HFNC) as alternative support methods. It is important to note that HFNC may not be sufficient and progression to NIV may be needed. Medical decisions should not be based only on survival; it is essential to consider the quality of life of the patient.

There are still many issues to resolve concerning intubation of end stage cancer patients and patients with hematologic malignancies. Because of legislations physicians may run into many ethical dilemmas whether to continue a futile support for a patient and delay the inevitable. There are many obstacles and dilemmas that physicians must overcome everyday concerning terminal stage patients with malignancies.

Keywords: intensive care unit, non-invasive ventilation, high-flow nasal cannula, malignancies, DNI

Introduction

Cancer management and treatment procedures are constantly advancing with newer chemotherapeutic agents, evolved surgical techniques as well as more targeted treatments against. Although newer treatments may be beneficial to patients, it can lead to compromised immune system increasing the likelihood of multiple organ dysfunction especially respiratory disorders. It is estimated that 40% of patients will suffer from respiratory failure and although the survival of cancer patients undergoing invasive mechanical ventilation (IMV) has improved, for some cancer patients, the institution of IMV is just an exercise of medical futility and prolongation of suffering [1]. Medical doctors often need to decide whether intubation will benefit ill terminal cancer patients.

However, there is only a small percentage of patients with directives and decisions concerning a do-not-intubate (DNI) order leaving the physicians with a difficult choice and ethical dilemmas. It is important to understand that refusing intubation is different from refusing resuscitation and the patients must be kept informed about their options and the impact of their decision. Patients may receive treatment and have resuscitation performed on them, if necessary, with respiratory support without intubation. In a DNR scenario the patient will not receive resuscitation only comfort measures.

Intubation and admission in the Intensive Care Unit (ICU) could be beneficial for some patients since it could provide them with the time to recover some of their respiratory function. Nowadays there is a better selection of patients that may benefit from mechanical ventilation and admission in the ICU.

While intubation and invasive mechanical ventilation is a cornerstone of supportive treatment for acute respiratory failure, a proportion of patients do not receive invasive mechanical ventilation due to factors such as patient preference for no intubation, physician belief that intubation would not offer any therapeutic benefit, or lack of resource availability resulting in triaging ICU beds and ventilators to other patients [2]. Intensive care units and other high-technology labor-intensive hospital services have come under increased pressure to contain their costs while maintaining the delivery of high-quality medical care [3]. Therefore, it is important that resources are not spent carelessly on patients that will not benefit from ICU admission and invasive mechanical ventilation.

Mortality Rates

Overall cancer death rates continue to decrease in both men and women for all major racial and ethnic groups. Overall cancer death rates from 2010 to 2014 decreased by 1.8% (95% confidence interval [CI] = –1.8% to –1.8%) per year in men, by 1.4% (95% CI = –1.4% to –1.3%) per year in women, and by 1.6% (95% CI = –2.0% to –1.3%) per year in children [4]. It is also noteworthy that recent progress in the treatment of many hematologic malignancies has resulted in improved population level 10-year survival, particularly chronic myeloid leukaemia (CML), chronic lymphocytic leukaemia (CLL), multiple myeloma (MM) [5].

The reduced mortality rates observed are contributed to few main reasons. First, advances in the treatment of solid tumors and hematologic malignancies produced a 20% decrease in overall mortality [6]. Secondly, there has been evolvement in the patient selection that will benefit from admission in the ICU. Finally, an earlier admission to the ICU has resulted in better survival rates for critically ill cancer patients [7].

Overall death rates due to cancer are decreasing for most types of cancer, indicating advancements in treatment but also the importance of prevention and early diagnosis. Despite this, the mortality remains high and medical decisions should not be based only on survival; it is essential to consider the quality of life of the patient. Many of the terminal stage patients do not want to spend their remaining time connected to a ventilator.

Alternatives to Endotracheal Intubation

Many patients with end-stage cancer that do not want futile treatment and procedures towards their end of life can sign legal orders such as do-not-intubate or do-not-resuscitate. Life and death decisions, including choices for Cardiopulmonary Resuscitation (CPR), in patients with cancer are complex and require a working knowledge of the patient's underlying disease, functional status, and, most important, his or her wishes concerning the level of care [8].

The aim of treatment and support as well as the expected end-results of will vary notably depending on the patient's such as a DNI order, or a comfort-measures only. When simple oxygen mask will not suffice, the physician must support the patient with alternative ways to provide maximal comfort and as little stress as possible. Such alternatives for intubation include non-invasive ventilation (NIV) and high-flow nasal cannula (HFNC).

Non-Invasive Ventilation

Mechanical ventilation without the use of an invasive artificial airway is defined as Non-Invasive Ventilation. Non-invasive positive-pressure ventilation (NPPV) using a mask (or interface) that conducts gas from a positive-pressure ventilator into the airways has become the predominant means of administering NIV [9]. In cases of a DNI order, the physician may use NIV as an alternative to intubation to support the patient's respiratory function.

Mortality is high among patients with hematologic malignancies admitted to intensive care units for acute respiratory failure [10]. Early management with non-invasive mechanical ventilation (NIMV) seems to improve outcomes and may even eliminate the need for ICU admission [11].

It is important that NIV offers an important ethical advantage for patients with hematologic malignancies, as it allows treatment of patients who refuse endotracheal intubation but not ventilatory support, thus permitting the delivery of intensive treatment while respecting the patients' will [12]. The use of NIV provides a level of relief for the patients from the stressful feeling and discomfort caused by respiratory failure.

High-Flow Nasal Cannula

High-flow nasal cannula therapy is an oxygen supply system capable of delivering up to 100% humidified and heated oxygen at a flow rate of up to 60 liters per minute [13]. The high flow rates will displace carbon dioxide in the physiological dead space (CO_2) and replace it with oxygen (O_2) with the prospect of improving oxygenation.

The main objective is to provide comfort to the patient; this is achieved by the heated and humidified administration of oxygen that reduces mucosal drying and irritation of the nasal passages leading to better cooperation and tolerance from the patient. In addition to the ability to generate high flow and concentration of supplemental oxygen, HFNC generates a low level of positive airway pressure, especially with the mouth closed [14].

When a patient is hypoxemic, the use of HFNC might prove advantageous over NIV since it can provide the support needed for the patient and supply adequate oxygenation while being more comfortable without the tight pressure from NIV mask. Another advantage of HFNC over NIV is that it requires less training to use. However, it is important to notice that HFNC may not be sufficient and progression to NIV may be needed. This progression is usually subjective for the physician based on both laboratory and clinical findings as well as the physician's expertise and experience.

Discussion

ARF is a leading cause of ICU admission among patients with hematologic malignancies or solid tumors [15]. Several patients may benefit from early intubation and mechanical ventilation while in other patients it proves to be futile. The patient and relatives should be informed about the possible complications of the treatment as well as the life expectancy of the patient and possibly make decisions about their end-of-life wishes.

Non-invasive ventilation has been used as an alternative for invasive ventilation in many scenarios, which renders it a valuable method especially when endotracheal intubation is against the patient's wishes. Both NIV and high-flow nasal cannula may be used to facilitate respiration and provide some relief in patients with DNI order; the physician must be familiar and have experience with these methods in order for them to be used as an alternative to intubation. It is also essential for the physician to be able to determine whether there is a place for NIV or negative implications surpass the potential benefits and affect the quality of life and comfort.

There are still many issues to resolve concerning intubation of end stage cancer patients and patients with hematologic malignancies. Physicians must be trained to better understand and recognize patients that will or will not benefit from intubation and ICU admission. Furthermore, there are different laws and procedures between countries, most of which do not include an official DNI option for patients forcing the doctors to resuscitate the patient.

Because of legislation, a physician will run into many ethical dilemmas whether to continue a futile support for a patient and delay the inevitable regardless of a Do-Not-Intubate order. To make matters worse, very often the relatives insist on intubation due to wrong impressions that intubation always saves lives and does not cause any harm even if it is against the patient's wishes putting the physician in an uncomfortable position. Additionally, there is the economic aspect to consider; resources should be used correctly since they are extremely limited in many medical centers and avoid wasting them in futile cases.

There are many obstacles and dilemmas that physicians must overcome everyday concerning terminal stage patients with malignancies. Patients and relatives must be educated and informed correctly about their condition and the course of action as well as their choice concerning the end of life. Doctors must be trained appropriately to be prepared when encountering these situations with terminally ill cancer patients. In our personal opinions, DNI and DNR orders must be allowed in more countries in order to avoid prolonging the suffering of the patient and allow them for a death with comfort and dignity.

Conclusion

ARF is a leading cause of ICU admission among patients with hematologic malignancies or solid tumors. Non-Invasive Ventilation and High-flow nasal cannula can be used as alternatives to intubation when a DNI order exists. It is essential to consider the quality of life of the patient and medical decisions should not be based only on survival. There are still many issues to resolve concerning intubation of end stage cancer patients and patients with hematologic malignancies. We need to avoid prolonging the suffering of the patient and allow them for a death with comfort and dignity.

References

[1] Huaringa, A. J., & Francis, W. H. (2018). Outcome of invasive mechanical ventilation in cancer patients: Intubate or not to intubate a patient with cancer. *Journal of Critical Care*. doi:10.1016/j.jcrc.2018.11.014.

[2] Wilson M E, Mittal A, Karki B, Dobler C C, Wahab A, Curtis J R, Erwin P J, Majzoub A M, Montori V M, Gajic O, Murad M H. Do-not-intubate orders in patients with acute respiratory failure: a systematic review and meta-analysis. *Intensive Care Med.* 2020 Jan;46(1):36-45. doi: 10.1007/s00134-019-05828-2. Epub 2019 Oct 28. PMID: 31659387; PMCID: PMC7223954.

[3] Kongsgaard U E, Meidell N K. Mechanical ventilation in critically ill cancer patients: outcome and utilisation of resources. *Support Care Cancer.* 1999 Mar;7 (2):95-9. doi: 10.1007/s005200050234. PMID: 10089090.

[4] Ahmedin Jemal, Elizabeth M Ward, Christopher J Johnson, Kathleen A Cronin, Jiemin Ma, A Blythe Ryerson, Angela Mariotto, Andrew J Lake, Reda Wilson, Recinda L Sherman, Robert N Anderson, S Jane Henley, Betsy A Kohler, Lynne Penberthy, Eric J Feuer, Hannah K Weir, Annual Report to the Nation on the Staqertus of Cancer, 1975–2014, Featuring Survival, *JNCI: Journal of the National Cancer Institute*, Volume 109, Issue 9, September 2017, djx030, https://doi.org/10.1093/jnci/djx030

[5] Pulte, D., Jansen, L. & Brenner, H. Changes in long term survival after diagnosis with common hematologic malignancies in the early 21st century. *Blood Cancer J.* 10, 56 (2020). https://doi.org/10.1038/s41408-020-0323-4.

[6] Brenner H. Long-term survival rates of cancer patients achieved by the end of the 20th century: a period analysis. *Lancet.* 2002; 360: 1131-1135.

[7] Anisoglou S, Asteriou C, Barbetakis N, Kakolyris S, Anastasiadou G, Pnevmatikos I. Outcome of lung cancer patients admitted to the intensive care unit with acute respiratory failure. *Hippokratia*. 2013;17(1):60-63.

[8] American Journal of Hospice & Palliative Medicine® Volume 24 Number 3 June/July 2007 224-229 © 2007 Sage Publications 10.1177/1049909107301485.

[9] Yamauchi LY, Travaglia TC, Bernardes SR, Figueiroa MC, Tanaka C, Fu C. Noninvasive positive-pressure ventilation in clinical practice at a large university-affiliated Brazilian hospital. *Clinics (Sao Paulo)*. 2012;67(7):767-772. doi:10.6061/clinics/2012(07)11.

[10] Gristina, G. R., Antonelli, M., Conti, G., Ciarlone, A., Rogante, S., Rossi, C., & Bertolini, G. (2011). Noninvasive versus invasive ventilation for acute respiratory failure in patients with hematologic malignancies: A 5-year multicenter observational survey. *Critical Care Medicine*, 39(10), 2232–2239. doi:10.1097/ccm.0b 013e3182227a27.

[11] Depuydt P O, Benoit D D, Vandewoude K H, Decruyenaere J M, Colardyn F A. Outcome in noninvasively and invasively ventilated hematologic patients with acute respiratory failure. *Chest.* 2004 Oct;126(4):1299-306. doi: 10.1378/chest.126.4.1299. PMID: 15486396.

[12] Meduri G U, Fox R C, Abou-Shala N, Leeper K V, Wunderink R G. Noninvasive mechanical ventilation via face mask in patients with acute respiratory failure who

refused endotracheal intubation. *Crit. Care Med.* 1994 Oct;22(10):1584-90. PMID: 7924369.

[13] Sharma S, Danckers M, Sanghavi D, Chakraborty R K. *High Flow Nasal Cannula.* 2022 Sep 21. In: StatPearls [Internet]. Treasure Island (FL): StatPearls Publishing; 2022 Jan–. PMID: 30252327./.

[14] Parke R, McGuinness S, Eccleston M. Nasal high-flow therapy delivers low level positive airway pressure. *Br. J. Anaesth.* 2009;103(6): 886-890.

[15] Azoulay É, Thiéry G, Chevret S, Moreau D, Darmon M, Bergeron A, Yang K, Meignin V, Ciroldi M, Le Gall J R, Tazi A, Schlemmer B. The prognosis of acute respiratory failure in critically ill cancer patients. *Medicine (Baltimore).* 2004 Nov;83(6):360-370. doi: 10.1097/01.md.0000145370.63676.fb. PMID: 15525848.

Chapter 18

Post Surgical Respiratory Failure (Cardiothoracic Surgery, Abdominal Surgery, Lung Resection)

Erdoğan Duran*, MD
Harran University Medical Faculty,
Department of Anesthesiology and Reanimation, Şanlıurfa, Turkey

Abstract

Postoperative hypoxemia/acute respiratory failure usually develops after abdominal and/or thoracic surgery. Postoperative pulmonary complications contribute significantly to postoperative morbidity and mortality. Postoperative respiratory failure has many causes, the prognosis and treatment of which differ. Preoperative clinical condition of the patient, localization of the surgical area, residual effects of anesthetics and muscle relaxants, agents that depress the respiratory center, postoperative pain are some of them.

The most important cause of acute respiratory failure in patients extubated after surgery, especially after upper abdominal and thoracic surgery, is the decrease in lung volumes with diaphragm dysfunction and atelectasis [1]. Oxygen administration is the first-line treatment in patients with acute respiratory failure. Non-invasive ventilation (NIV) and high flow nasal cannula (HFNC) can be used in addition to conventional face and nasal oxygen masks to ensure adequate tissue oxygenation without re-intubation of patients.

Invasive mechanical ventilation is used as supportive therapy in patients where these methods cannot improve oxygenation. NIV can usually be administered with positive end-expiratory airway pressure

* Corresponding Author's Email: drerdoganduran6331@gmail.com.

In: Nasal High Flow and Non-Invasive Ventilatory Support
Editors: A. M. Esquinas, D. A. Lagonidis, P. Silva Santos et al.
ISBN: 979-8-88697-420-1

(PEEP), continuous positive airway pressure (CPAP), or bilevel positive airway pressure (BIPAP). HFNC can produce a slight positive pressure increase at the end of expiration [2]. In this section, the escalation approach in the management of oxygen therapy will be emphasized, especially in respiratory failure after cardiothoracic surgery, abdominal surgery and lung resection.

Keywords: non-invasive ventilation, high-flow nasal cannula, cardiothoracic surgery, abdominal surgery, lung resection

Introduction

Despite advances in invasive mechanical ventilation therapy, the risk of reintubation in the first 96-hours after extubation postoperatively is approximately 10-15%. This frequency may vary in different studies according to the patient and many risk factors. Reintubation is associated with morbidity and mortality. In order to provide oxygenation after extubation and reduce reintubation, oxygen support with conventional methods and respiratory support with NIV or HFNC are applied [3].

Oxygen is traditionally delivered via low-flow systems such as nasal cannulas or masks, or high-flow systems such as Venturi masks. Such conventional systems do not deliver a significant portion of the inspired oxygen, and often prolonged use cannot be tolerated due to insufficient heating and humidification of the inspired gas.

NIV is a means of providing mechanical oxygenation in the non-intubated patient. In clinical practice, ventilation is provided with positive end-expiratory airway pressure (PEEP) and pressure support. In pressure support, the peak pressure can be increased up to a maximum of 20 cmH_2O. At higher pressures, air leakage from the mask generally occurs and limits the pressure build-up above these values. Although NIV is beneficial initially, it may not be sufficient to meet the respiratory workload with the progression of the underlying disease.

Oxygen delivery via HFNC has a number of differences from conventional methods. These differences include small flexible nasal tips, warming and humidifying oxygen, flushing the nasopharyngeal dead space, continuous positive airway pressure (CPAP) effect, high flow rates (usually > 40 Lmin), reduced inspiratory effort. It is thought that all of these increase oxygenation by reducing the work of breathing and provide better patient comfort [4].

Cardiothoracic Surgery

Postoperative pulmonary complications are common after cardiothoracic surgery. However, its incidence in the literature varies widely according to the preoperative condition of the patients and the surgery to be performed. Alveolar collapse or atelectasis is one of the most important problems in extubated patients after cardiothoracic surgery. These complications cause prolonged hospital stays, increased morbidity and hospital costs [5].

NIV is frequently used in specific patient groups to prevent complications and treat acute respiratory failure. In a study published by Zarbock et al. NIV after cardiac surgery was shown to significantly reduce pulmonary complications [6].

In another, retrospective analysis of 63 patients with respiratory failure who underwent NIV after cardiac surgery, it was stated that NIV failed within 24 hours and mortality could be reduced by early intubation in some patients [7].

Few studies in children suggest that NIV may be safe and valuable in the treatment of hypoxemic or hypercapnic acute respiratory failure after cardiac surgery. It has been reported that HFNC has fewer complications compared to NIV/BiPAP in preventing post-extubation respiratory failure in patients who have undergone pediatric cardiac surgery [8].

With the technological developments in recent years, the use of HFNC has become more and more widespread. In a larger study comparing NIV and HFNC, NIV and HFNC had similar reintubation and mortality rates after cardiothoracic surgery. Due to its' comfortable and tolerabl features HFNC can be used as an alternative therapy to NIV [9].

In a meta-analysis, it was stated that the use of HFNC in the postoperative period immediately after cardiothoracic surgery reduces reintubation compared to conventional oxygen therapy. Furthermore, the findings support the use of postoperative prophylactic HFNC in high-risk and/or obese patients undergoing cardiothoracic surgery [10].

Although studies on the use of HFNC after cardiothoracic surgery have increased, the clinical condition of the patient and the clinician's experience will be decisive in the choice of HFNC.

Lung Resection

Thoracic surgery patients are at the highest risk of developing postoperative pulmonary complications after surgery. Although advances in anesthesia have improved perioperative and postoperative care, pulmonary complications after lung resection remain the leading causes of death [9].

Positive pressure applied with the use of NIV in thoracic surgery patients may cause air leakage at the lung resection site. However, there are few studies on this subject [9].

In a study comparing conventional oxygen therapy and NIV after lung resection, it was stated that NIV reduced the need for postoperative mechanical ventilation and in-hospital mortality. However, the risk factors for long-term NIV failure are unclear [11]. It is stated that NIV may be an alternative to conventional ventilation, even after higher-risk lung transplantation and esophagectomy surgeries [12]. In the presence of expert personnel and sufficient technological equipment, NIV is recommended to prevent/treat respiratory failure after lung resection. However, the risks of positive pressure should be considered [13].

Although data on the use of HFNC after lung resection is limited, it has been considered as an alternative to conventional oxygen therapy and NIV in eligible patients. A recent study, which compares HFNC and venturi mask after thoracotomy lung resection, demonstrated HFNC did not reduce the incidence of postoperative hypoxemia. Further studies are needed to determine whether HFNC can provide clinical benefit on carbon dioxide clearance, postoperative hypoxemia, and pulmonary complications [13].

Abdominal Surgery

There may be many reasons for the development of hypoxemia in the immediate post-operative period. Similar to cardiothoracic surgery, postoperative pain in abdominal surgeries close to the diaphragm may cause atelectasis due to diaphragmatic dysfunction. The residual depressing effect of anesthetic agents can also cause hypoxia with a decrease in lung capacity. Postoperative pulmonary complications decrease as the incision moves away from the diaphragm in abdominal surgeries. Except for low-flow oxygen, there is no single treatment method routinely used to prevent or treat postoperative acute respiratory failure in this population. Other options include NIV and

HFNC [1, 14]. Besides analgesia, NIV oxygen therapy with an appropriate pressure will usually be sufficient to correct hypoxemia.

Continuous positive airway pressure may be beneficial in patients without profuse secretions. In patients with hypoxemic respiratory failure following abdominal surgery, the use of NIV has reduced the risk of tracheal reintubation compared to standard oxygen therapy. These findings support the use of NIV in this setting [14]. In a recent study by Jaber et al., it was reported that the use of NIV reduced reintubation, hospital stay, and mortality compared to conventional therapy in patients with respiratory failure after abdominal surgery [14].

In a recent meta-analysis supporting that the use of NIV in the post-abdominal surgery period can increase lung aeration and reduce the amount of atelectasis, it was stated that HFNC also prevents intubation in acute hypoxic respiratory failure compared to conventional oxygen therapy. The reintubation rate and respiratory therapy failure of HFNC were not different from NIV. However, data examining the routine use of HFNC in the early postoperative period are not very clear [10].

Conclusion

In order to prevent respiratory failure that may develop in the early postoperative period, the clinical condition of the patient should be evaluated in the preoperative period and necessary precautions should be taken. If respiratory complications develop in the postoperative period, treatment should be planned depending on the cause, intubation should be avoided first by providing gas exchange, via conventional oxygen delivery methods, NIV, HFNC, which can be used depending on the patient's condition. When necessary, it should not be too late for invasive mechanical ventilation. Patient selection should be done carefully, especially in high-risk cardiothoracic surgery and abdominal surgery patient population if NIV is to be preferred in the treatment of postoperative respiratory failure.

There is a wealth of data showing that NIV is safer and more effective in preventing desaturation than standard oxygen therapy in this group of patients. The opinions that NIV can be used effectively to improve oxygenation and reduce atelectasis by ventilating the lungs without disturbing hemodynamics are more dominant. It has been shown that the use of NIV in different modes, depending on the clinical condition of the patient, reduces the rates of hospital stay, hospital-acquired pneumonia, morbidity, mortality, and reintubation in patients undergoing abdominal surgery, thoracic surgery, and cardiac surgery. The use of NIV is recommended in acute respiratory failure. Further clinical studies are also needed for more detailed evaluations.

It has been observed that HFNC does not increase reintubation rates compared to NIV in abdominal surgeries near the diaphragm and surgeries above the diaphragm. Although there are studies supporting that HFNC can be an alternative to NIV, the use of HFNC should be supported by comprehensive studies, especially in risky patient groups. In acute respiratory failure after lung resection, positive pressure should be optimized in the use of NIV. If HFNC is to be preferred in this patient group, HFNC should be adjusted according to the patient's condition and followed closely by experienced personnel. However, both applications should be supported by larger clinical studies.

References

[1] Rochwerg, B., Brochard, L., Elliott, M. W., Hess, D., Hill, N. S., Nava, S., Navalesi, P., Antonelli, M., Brozek, J., Conti, G., Ferrer, M., Guntupalli, K., Jaber, S., Keenan, S., Mancebo, J., Mehta, S., Raoof, S.: Official ERS/ATS clinical practice guidelines: noninvasive ventilation for acute respiratory failure. *Eur. Respir. J.* 50, 1602426 (2017). https://doi.org/10.1183/13993003.02426-2016.

[2] Spoletini, G., Alotaibi, M., Blasi, F., Hill, N. S.: Heated Humidified High-Flow Nasal Oxygen in Adults. *Chest.* 148, 253–261 (2015). https://doi.org/10.1378/chest.14-2871.

[3] Casey, J. D., Vaughan, E. R., Lloyd, B. D., Bilas, P. A., Hall, E. J., Toporek, A. H., Buell, K. G., Brown, R. M., Richardson, R. K., Rooks, J. C., Wang, L., Lindsell, C. J., Ely, E. W., Self, W. H., Bernard, G. R., Rice, T. W., Semler, M. W.: Protocolized Post-Extubation Respiratory Support to prevent reintubation: protocol and statistical analysis plan for a clinical trial. *BMJ Open.* 9, e030476 (2019). https://doi.org/10.1136/bmjopen-2019-030476.

[4] Rittayamai, N., Tscheikuna, J., Rujiwit, P.: High-Flow Nasal Cannula Versus Conventional Oxygen Therapy After Endotracheal Extubation: A Randomized Crossover Physiologic Study. *Respir. Care.* 59, 485–490 (2014). https://doi.org/10.4187/respcare.02397.

[5] Joshi, P., Fraser, J. F., Mullany, D. V.: The high risk cardiac surgical patient. *Curr. Anaesth. Crit. Care.* 16, 369–383 (2005). https://doi.org/10.1016/j.cacc.2006.05.001.

[6] Zarbock, A., Mueller, E., Netzer, S., Gabriel, A., Feindt, P., Kindgen-Milles, D.: Prophylactic Nasal Continuous Positive Airway Pressure Following Cardiac Surgery Protects From Postoperative Pulmonary Complications. *Chest.* 135, 1252–1259 (2009). https://doi.org/10.1378/chest.08-1602.

[7] García-Delgado, M., Navarrete, I., García-Palma, M. J., Colmenero, M.: Postoperative Respiratory Failure After Cardiac Surgery: Use of Noninvasive Ventilation. *J. Cardiothorac. Vasc. Anesth*. 26, 443–447 (2012). https://doi.org/10.1053/j.jvca.2011.11.007.

[8] Jayashankar, J., Rajan, P., Kottayil, B., Jayant, A., Balachandran, R.: Comparison of nasal bi-level positive airway pressure versus high-flow nasal cannula as a means of noninvasive respiratory support in pediatric cardiac surgery. *Anesth. Essays Res*. 14, 283 (2020). https://doi.org/10.4103/aer.AER_39_20.

[9] Stéphan, F., Barrucand, B., Petit, P., Rézaiguia-Delclaux, S., Médard, A., Delannoy, B., Cosserant, B., Flicoteaux, G., Imbert, A., Pilorge, C., Bérard, L.: High-Flow Nasal Oxygen vs Noninvasive Positive Airway Pressure in Hypoxemic Patients After Cardiothoracic Surgery. *JAMA*. 313, 2331 (2015). https://doi.org/10.1001/jama.2015.5213.

[10] Chaudhuri, D., Granton, D., Wang, D. X., Burns, K. E. A., Helviz, Y., Einav, S., Trivedi, V., Mauri, T., Ricard, J.-D., Mancebo, J., Frat, J.-P., Jog, S., Hernandez, G., Maggiore, S. M., Mbuagbaw, L., Hodgson, C. L., Jaber, S., Goligher, E. C., Brochard, L., Rochwerg, B.: High-Flow Nasal Cannula in the Immediate Postoperative Period. *Chest*. 158, 1934–1946 (2020). https://doi.org/10.1016/j.chest.2020.06.038.

[11] Auriant, I., Jallot, A., Hervé, P., Cerrina, J., Le Roy Ladurie, F., Fournier, J. L., Lescot, B., Parquin, F.: Noninvasive Ventilation Reduces Mortality in Acute Respiratory Failure following Lung Resection. *Am. J. Respir. Crit. Care Med*. 164, 1231–1235 (2001). https://doi.org/10.1164/ajrccm.164.7.2101089.

[12] Rocco, M., Conti, G., Antonelli, M., Bufi, M., Costa, M., Alampi, D., Ruberto, F., Stazi, G., Pietropaoli, P.: Non-invasive pressure support ventilation in patients with acute respiratory failure after bilateral lung transplantation. *Intensive Care Med*. 27, 1622–1626 (2001). https://doi.org/10.1007/s001340101063.

[13] Pennisi, M. A., Bello, G., Congedo, M. T., Montini, L., Nachira, D., Ferretti, G. M., Meacci, E., Gualtieri, E., De Pascale, G., Grieco, D. L., Margaritora, S., Antonelli, M.: Early nasal high-flow versus Venturi mask oxygen therapy after lung resection: a randomized trial. *Crit. Care*. 23, 68 (2019). https://doi.org/10.1186/s13054-019-2361-5.

[14] Jaber, S., Lescot, T., Futier, E., Paugam-Burtz, C., Seguin, P., Ferrandiere, M., Lasocki, S., Mimoz, O., Hengy, B., Sannini, A., Pottecher, J., Abback, P.-S., Riu, B., Belafia, F., Constantin, J.-M., Masseret, E., Beaussier, M., Verzilli, D., De Jong, A., Chanques, G., Brochard, L., Molinari, N.: Effect of Noninvasive Ventilation on Tracheal Reintubation Among Patients With Hypoxemic Respiratory Failure Following Abdominal Surgery. *JAMA*. 315, 1345 (2016). https://doi.org/10.1001/jama.2016.2706.

Chapter 19

Acute Hypoxemic Respiratory Failure during Bronchoscopy

Diana Pimenta*, MD
and Rui Rolo, MD
Pulmonology Department, Braga Hospital, Braga, Portugal

Abstract

Flexible bronchoscopy is a safe and frequently performed procedure for the assessment, diagnosis, and treatment of patients with respiratory illnesses. The insertion of a flexible bronchoscope into the airway decreases the cross-sectional area proportional to the outside diameter of the bronchoscope and increases the resistance to airflow. During flexible bronchoscopy, the arterial oxygen partial pressure may drop, increasing the risk of respiratory failure.

To avoid episodes of desaturation during the procedure, several oxygenation strategies have been proposed, including conventional oxygen therapy, high-flow nasal cannula oxygen therapy (HFNC), continuous positive airway pressure (CPAP), and non-invasive ventilation (NIV). Non-invasive ventilation (NIV) with continuous positive pressure or intermittent positive pressure is a safe and effective means of recruiting alveoli and increasing ventilation in patients with acute respiratory failure, being well tolerated and associated with a low rate of complications. HFNC consists of a mixture of air and oxygen, delivered from a heated and humidified maximum flow of up to 60 L/min, and has been used successfully to prevent the worsening of acute respiratory failure during bronchoscopy.

---

* Corresponding Author's Email: dianapimenta.hb@gmail.com.

In: Nasal High Flow and Non-Invasive Ventilatory Support
Editors: A. M. Esquinas, D. A. Lagonidis, P. Silva Santos et al.
ISBN: 979-8-88697-420-1

The oxygenation strategy during flexible bronchoscopy in a patient with hypoxemic acute respiratory failure should be chosen according to the procedure, pulmonary and cardiac function, oxygen requirement during the procedure and risk of acute respiratory failure.

Keywords: bronchoscopy, acute respiratory failure, non-invasive ventilation, high-flow nasal cannula oxygen therapy

Respiratory Physiology during Bronchoscopy

Flexible bronchoscopy is a safe and frequently performed procedure for the assessment, diagnosis, and treatment of patients with respiratory illnesses. The procedure and its applications have evolved progressively since its introduction in 1968. Nowadays, flexible bronchoscopy is an essential diagnostic and therapeutic tool in respiratory medicine and an increasingly important and well-tolerated procedure that can be safely performed in an outpatient setting [1]. It allows direct visualization of the upper and lower airways through an optical fiber that contains a light source and video at its distal end. In addition to being a safe procedure, it has a high diagnostic yield, particularly in situations of hemoptysis, respiratory infection, parenchymal and interstitial lung diseases, pulmonary nodules or masses, persistent pulmonary infiltrates, mediastinal adenopathies, suspected rejection of lung transplantation, among others.

Regarding therapeutic indications, it is extremely useful in cases of foreign body aspiration, ablation or cytoreduction of endobronchial lesions, airway stenosis and lung lavage [1, 2, 3]. The most common adverse events include tachycardia, bradycardia, hemorrhage, bronchospasm, laryngospasm, cough, dyspnea, odynophagia, apnea, seizure, desaturation, pneumothorax, and pulmonary edema. The rate of serious complications described in the literature is around 1.1%, with a mortality rate of 0.02%. [1, 3, 4]. Most patients undergoing flexible bronchoscopy have conditions that impair gas exchange, such as pneumonia, interstitial lung diseases, lung cancer, and endobronchial lesions [2].

The insertion of a flexible bronchoscope into the airway decreases the cross-sectional area proportional to the outside diameter of the bronchoscope and increases the resistance to airflow.

In non-intubated patients, the fiberscope occupies approximately 10% of the cross-sectional area of the trachea and 15% of the cricoid ring. This aspect, normally irrelevant in patients without hypoxemia, can be harmful in a hypoxemic patient, as it not only increases the work of breathing, but also decreases the PaO_2 by 10-20 mm Hg after an uncomplicated bronchoscopy. Hypoxemia is commonly seen during bronchoscopy and is multifactorial. It is related to patient sedation, fiberscope passage through the vocal cords, patient positioning and intra-procedural sampling [1, 2, 3]. In addition, aspiration during bronchoscopy reduces end-expiratory lung volume, causing alveolar collapse, impairing ventilation-perfusion, and so increasing the risk of respiratory failure [2]. The time interval to normalization of gas exchange after bronchoscopy varies from 15 minutes for normal lungs to several hours in patients with severe alterations in the lung parenchyma [2, 3].

Monitoring patients using pulse oximetry during bronchoscopy is an accurate non-invasive method to assess hypoxemia. Most desaturations are transient and do not require specific intervention [2].

Flexible Bronchoscopy in the Patient with Hypoxemic Acute Respiratory Failure: Therapeutic Strategies

As already mentioned, during flexible bronchoscopy the arterial oxygen partial pressure may drop, increasing the risk of respiratory failure. To avoid episodes of desaturation during the procedure, several oxygenation strategies have been proposed, including conventional oxygen therapy, high flow nasal cannula oxygen therapy (HFNC), continuous positive airway pressure (CPAP), and non-invasive ventilation (NIV). Nasal catheter oxygen therapy is appropriate to reduce transient hypoxemia. However, the inspired oxygen fraction (FiO_2) cannot be predicted and may not be sufficient in severe cases. When lung parenchyma is already compromised by an underlying pathological condition, flexible bronchoscopy can impair gas exchange, exacerbating respiratory failure [1, 2].

Some patients with acute respiratory failure require diagnostic or therapeutic bronchoscopy. Although bronchoscopy is considered a safe intervention, it is known that bronchoscopy, especially bronchoalveolar lavage (BAL) can induce significant hypoxemia. Thus, severe hypoxemia represents a contraindication to bronchoscopy if it cannot be reversed by therapeutic interventions. In these patients, the benefits of the procedure must be weighed against the possible risks [4].

Non-Invasive Ventilation (NIV)

Non-invasive ventilation (NIV) with continuous positive pressure or intermittent positive pressure is a safe and effective means of recruiting alveoli and increasing ventilation in patients with acute respiratory failure, being well tolerated and associated with a low rate of complications. Thus, NIV is cornerstone in the treatment of acute respiratory failure of various etiologies [4, 5].

NIV used for preoxygenation is more effective in reducing arterial oxyhemoglobin desaturation than usual preoxygenation during orotracheal intubation in severely hypoxemic patients [3]. Continuous positive airway pressure (CPAP) has been studied during flexible bronchoscopy. CPAP therapy allows the maintenance of a positive pressure throughout the entire respiratory cycle, recruiting atelectatic regions of the lung, reducing venous mixing and decreasing the patient's inspiratory effort. Maitre et al., studied the use of CPAP through a face mask during flexible bronchoscopy in patients with hypoxemic acute respiratory failure (PaO_2 /FiO_2 <300 mmHg). In this study, CPAP therapy, in comparison to conventional oxygen therapy, ensured higher SpO_2 during and after the procedure, in addition to the fact that fewer patients needed ventilatory assistance in the 6 hours after the procedure [2, 5].

As mentioned above, in 1996, Antonelli et al., studied the use of NIV in immunocompromised patients with severe acute respiratory failure (PaO_2/ FiO_2 ratio < 100) [6].

The authors reported that NIV, applied 10 minutes before and discontinued 90 minutes after flexible bronchoscopy, was well tolerated and improved gas exchange the need for intubation. In 2002 they returned to study the use of NIV, but this time, in immunocompetent patients with acute respiratory failure, with less severe hypoxemia (PaO_2/FiO_2 ratio < 200) [6]. The study included 26 patients with a PaO_2/FiO_2 ratio < 200 who needed flexible bronchoscopy and bronchoalveolar lavage for suspected nosocomial pneumonia. Thirteen patients were randomized to receive conventional oxygen supplementation during the intervention and thirteen patients to the NIV group.

The authors found that during bronchoscopy, the mean PaO_2/FiO_2 ratio increased by 82% in the group of patients under NIV and decreased around 10% in the group of patients under supplemental O_2 by Venturi mask. Patients were evaluated approximately 60 minutes after bronchoscopy and the group of patients undergoing NIV was found to have a higher mean PaO_2/FiO_2 ratio and a lower mean heart rate than patients who underwent the examination under conventional oxygen therapy. Thus, the authors concluded that in patients with severe hypoxemia, NIV is superior to conventional oxygen therapy in preventing deterioration of gas exchange during flexible bronchoscopy, and with better hemodynamic tolerance [7].

In 2003, Antonelli et al., concluded that performing flexible bronchoscopy and BAL in patients with acute respiratory failure under NIV through a Helmet interface also allows for a safe diagnosis, preventing deterioration of gas exchange and, consequently, orotracheal intubation [8].

Bauman et al., in 2011, carried out a prospective observational cohort study in hospitalized patients with acute respiratory failure, who needed to undergo bronchoscopy, under NIV. In this study, during bronchoscopy, the inspiratory pressure was adjusted from 10 to 25 cmH_2O and the positive end-expiratory pressure (PEEP) from 5 to 10 cmH_2O, in order to obtain optimal ventilation and oxygenation [4].

A simple face mask, fitted to the patient' face using elastic straps, was used. A swivel connector (T adapter) was inserted between the ventilator tube and the mask to allow insertion of the fiberscope (Figure 1). The patient was sedated following clinical protocols (combination of 1 to 2 mg of midazolam and administration of 10 to 20 mg of intravenous propofol every 2 to 3 min). After bronchoscopy, all patients maintained non-invasive ventilatory support for at least 2 hours. The results obtained demonstrate a low rate of complications in this group of patients. Only four patients required endotracheal intubation during the first eight hours after bronchoscopy (10%), a result that is within the acceptable range. Therefore, bronchoscopy can be performed with an acceptable risk in patients with severe acute hypoxemic respiratory failure already on non-invasive ventilatory support. As these patients are at high risk of endotracheal intubation secondary to NIV failure, bronchoscopy should only be performed by physicians experienced in bronchoscopy and endotracheal intubation, in a high-level monitoring setting.

Early etiological diagnosis in critically ill patients is important for proper treatment. Baumann et al., showed that BAL during NIV provided diagnostic information in 68% of patients with acute respiratory failure [4].

In 2016, Korkmaz Ekren et al., carried out a prospective observational study whose objective was to assess the feasibility, safety, and contribution to the diagnosis and/or modification of the ongoing treatment, in view of the performance of flexible bronchoscopy in hospitalized patients diagnosed with acute respiratory distress syndrome (ARDS) under NIV treatment [9]. In this study, they used either an oro-nasal mask or a face mask adapted to a connector (bronchoscopy elbow, Philips Respironics) for the passage of the bronchoscope (Figure 2) [9].

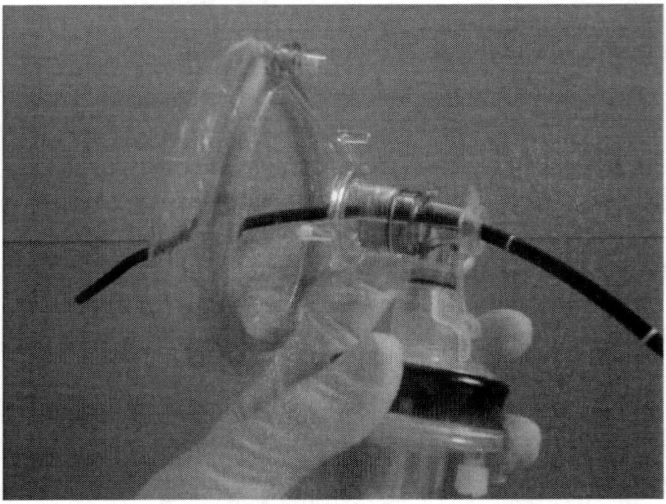

Figure 1. Bronchoscope inserted through swivel connector in face mask.

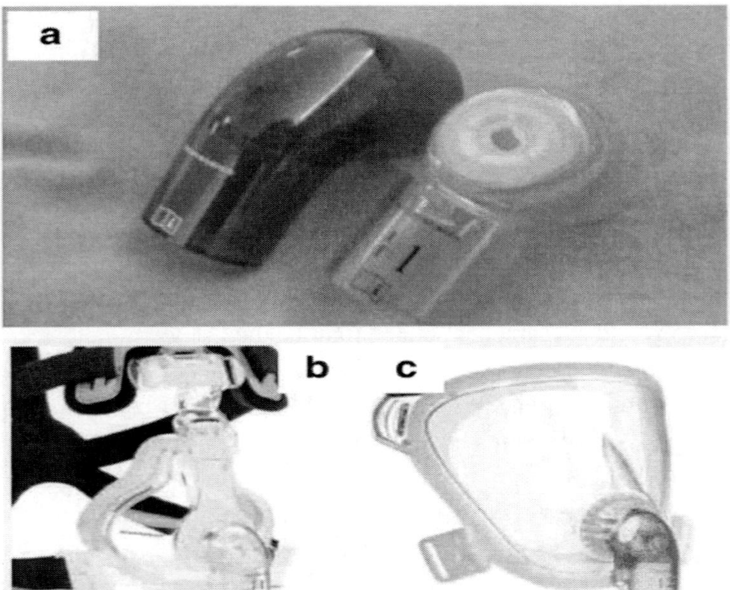

Figure 2. a - Connector used between the ventilator tube and the mask for the insertion of the flexible bronchoscope; b - Oronasal mask; c - Face mask.

The study demonstrated that bronchoscopy under NIV is feasible and safe, being an effective diagnostic and therapeutic procedure in patients with ARDS, and that it can be performed safely and without major complications in this group of patients.

The use of NIV during flexible bronchoscopy has been extended to other procedures, namely transbronchial lung biopsy. In this study, a group of 6 patients who had diffuse bilateral parenchymal infiltrates and $PaO_2/FiO_2 < 200$ mm Hg underwent bronchoscopy lung biopsy under NIV. NIV was started 10 minutes before the procedure and continued for 30 minutes after the end of the procedure [3].

During lung biopsy, CPAP was reduced to zero and only a pressure support of 10 cmH_2O was maintained. The procedure was well tolerated, and all patients maintained $SpO_2 > 92\%$ during the procedure. Only one patient required endotracheal intubation due to hemoptysis. Definitive diagnosis was obtained in 5 of the 6 patients. Also in another study, Scala et al., showed that in patients hospitalized for an acute exacerbation of COPD with hypercapnic encephalopathy due to community-acquired pneumonia and who were unable to expel secretions, the use of NIV during therapeutic bronchoscopy was associated with improvement in PaO_2/FIO_2 [10].

High-Flow Nasal Cannula Oxygen Therapy

High-Flow Nasal Cannula Oxygen Therapy (HFNC) consists of a mixture of air and oxygen, delivered through a maximum heated and humidified flow of up to 60 L/min. This strategy has been used successfully to prevent the worsening of acute respiratory failure during bronchoscopy [2].

Kim et al., conducted a study whose aim was to investigate the safety and efficacy of HFNC during bronchoscopy and BAL in patients with acute respiratory failure. The authors concluded that this therapy was effective and safe in patients with mild to moderate respiratory failure.

In this sense, Chung et al., carried out a retrospective study based on the performance of bronchoscopy in patients with hypoxemic acute respiratory failure under HFNC support. The authors demonstrated the clinical efficacy associated with the use of the HFNC during bronchoscopy in this group of patients. HFNC therapy helps to avoid mucosal damage and patient discomfort, as the oxygen supplied is humidified and warmed [2, 11].

Based on the studies carried out so far, it can be stated that HFNC surpasses conventional oxygen therapy in patients with mild to moderate respiratory failure. On the other hand, the data suggest the superiority of NIV in patients with more severe acute respiratory failure compared to HFNC [2].

Growing evidence in favor of high-flow cannula and NIV has generated some studies comparing both in patients with mild to moderate hypoxemic acute respiratory failure. Compared with high-flow cannula, NIV improved oxygenation prior to, during and after flexible bronchoscopy, as well as decreases the number of desaturations <90%, with no difference in mortality or in the rate of patients requiring invasive intubation and invasive mechanical ventilation [2].

Conclusion

The oxygenation strategy during flexible bronchoscopy in a patient with hypoxemic acute respiratory failure should be chosen according to the procedure, pulmonary and cardiac function, oxygen requirement during the procedure and risk of acute respiratory failure. In patients with mild to moderate need for oxygen, high-flow therapy is preferable to conventional oxygen therapy, whereas the use of CPAP or NIV is preferable in patients with more severe hypoxemia [2].

Although several studies have shown benefits of different oxygenation strategies during bronchoscopy in patients with acute respiratory failure, there are still no clear guidelines available in the literature. There remains a lack of evidence to make a clear recommendation on the use of one oxygenation strategy over another. Optimizing oxygenation during bronchoscopy remains an important safety issue for patients with acute respiratory failure undergoing this procedure.

References

[1] Du Rand A, Blaikley J, Booton R, Chaudhuri N, Gupta V, Khalid S, Mandal S, Martin J, Mills J, Navani N, Rahman N M, Wrightson J M, Munavvar M. "British Thoracic Society guideline for diagnostic flexible bronchoscopy in adults." *Thorax*, 2013: i1–i44.

[2] Pelaia C, Bruni A, Garofalo E, Rovida S, Arrighi E, Cammarota G, Navalesi P, Pelaia G, Longhini F. "Oxygenation strategies during fexible bronchoscopy: a review of the literature." *Respir. Res*., 2021: 1-13.

[3] Ritesh Agarwal, Ajmal Khan, Ashutosh N Aggarwal, Dheeraj Gupta. "Bronchoscopic Lung Biopsy Using Noninvasive Ventilatory Support: Case Series

and Review of Literature of NIV-Assisted Bronchoscopy." *Respiratory Care*, 2012: 1927-1936.

[4] Hans Jörg Baumann, Hans Klose, Marcel Simon, Tarik Ghadban, Stephan A Braune, Jan K Hennigs, Stefan Kluge. "Fiber optic bronchoscopy in patients with acute hypoxemic respiratory failure requiring noninvasive ventilation - a feasibility study." *Critical Care*, 2011: 1-7.

[5] Maitre B, Jaber S, Maggiore S M, Bergot E, Richard J C, Bakthiari H, Housset B, Boussignac G, Brochard L. "Continuous positive airway pressure during fiberoptic bronchoscopy in hypoxemic patients. A randomized double-blind study using a new device." *Am. J. Respir. Crit. Care Med.*, 2000: 1063–1067.

[6] Antonelli M, Conti G, Riccioni L, Meduri GU. "Noninvasive positive-pressure ventilation via face mask during bronchoscopy with BAL in high-risk hypoxemic patients." *Chest*, 1996: 724–728.

[7] Antonelli M, Conti G, Rocco M, Arcangeli A, Cavaliere F, Proietti R, Meduri GU. "Noninvasive positive-pressure ventilation vs conventional oxygen supplementation in hypoxemic patients undergoing diagnostic bronchoscopy." *Chest*, 2002: 1149–1154.

[8] Antonelli M, Pennisi M A, Conti G, Bello G, Maggiore S M, Michetti V, Cavaliere F, Proietti R. "Fiberoptic bronchoscopy during noninvasive positive pressure ventilation delivered by helmet." *Intensive Care Med.*, 2003: 126–129.

[9] Korkmaz Ekren P, Basarik Aydogan B, Gurgun A, Tasbakan M S, Bacakoglu F, Nava S. "Can fiberoptic bronchoscopy be applied to critically ill patients treated with noninvasive ventilation for acute respiratory distress syndrome? Prospective observational study." *BMC Pulm. Med.*, 2016: 1-8.

[10] Raffaele Scala, Mario Naldi, Uberto Maccari. "Early fiberoptic bronchoscopy during non-invasive ventilation in patients with decompensated chronic obstructive pulmonary disease due to community-acquired-pneumonia." *Critical Care*, 2010: 1-12.

[11] Chung S M, Choi J W, Lee Y S, Choi J H, Oh J Y, Min K H, Hur G Y, Lee S Y, Shim J J, Kang K H. "Clinical effectiveness of high-flow nasal cannula in hypoxaemic patients during bronchoscopic procedures." *Tuberc. Respir. Dis.*, 2019: 81-85.

Chapter 20

De-Escalation Therapy in Non-Invasive Ventilatory Approaches: Evidence and Tools for Health Care

Anaura Carrasquel R.[1,*], MD
Alexis Jaspe C.[2], MD
and Estefanía Perez M.[1], MD
[1] Emergency Department, Ramón y Cajal Hospital, Madrid, Spain
[2] Intensive Care Unit, Gregorio Marañón Hospital, Madrid, Spain

Abstract

Non-invasive mechanical ventilation and the use of high-flow oxygen therapy have been shown to be therapeutic tools highly effective in the treatment of certain respiratory pathologies. These are techniques with great repercussion in terms of cost benefit, since they reduce the days of hospitalization, as well as the need for orotracheal intubation and invasive mechanical ventilation, thus reducing the need for admission to Intensive Care Units as well as morbidity and mortality associated with admission of patients in these units.

Keywords: non-invasive ventilation, high-flow nasal cannula, acute respiratory failure, weaning, hypoxemia, de-escalation

---

[*] Corresponding Author's Email: carrasquelregalade@gmail.com.

In: Nasal High Flow and Non-Invasive Ventilatory Support
Editors: A. M. Esquinas, D. A. Lagonidis, P. Silva Santos et al.
ISBN: 979-8-88697-420-1

Introduction

Acute respiratory failure (ARF) is a common presentation to the emergency department. Oxygen therapy is a treatment in cases that involve hypoxia [1]. Non-invasive oxygenation strategies [high-flow nasal oxygen, non-invasive ventilation] compared with standard oxygen therapy have been shown to be capable of preventing endotracheal intubation in patients with mild hypoxemia [2].

Use of non-invasive oxygenation strategies preserves physiological pathways of airway protection (cough and clearance of secretions) [3] and may directly reduce the complications related to endotracheal intubation [e.g., laryngeal, and tracheal trauma] and invasive mechanical ventilation.

These include ventilator-induced lung injury, ventilator-associated pneumonia, sedation, and neuromuscular paralysis [4]. By preserving patients' alertness and interaction with the environment, use of non-invasive support reduces the risk of discomfort and delirium.

Early use of non-invasive ventilation is recommended because the opportunity for a successful start might be lost if delays arise and the patient's underlying disease progresses too far. However, such ventilation can be started too early—i.e., when the patient's illness is so mild that no ventilatory assistance is needed and they are more likely to be intolerant than be helped. Thus, judgment should be exercised; most practitioners seek evidence of increased dyspnea and work of breathing (tachypnoea or heightened accessory muscle use) [5].

Another advantage of an early start is that patients who are not in immediate life-threatening situations can be managed outside the intensive care units, provided that the ward team has the necessary skills. Hence specialized units (respiratory intensive care, high dependency) are ideal for provision of non-invasive ventilation to all but the sickest patients because they offer complete non-invasive monitoring systems and higher nurse to patient ratios than are available on general wards.

Benefits of Using High-Flow Nasal Prongs in Respiratory Failure

High-flow oxygen via nasal cannula rapidly alleviates symptoms of acute respiratory failure and improves oxygenation by several mechanisms, including dead space washout, reduction in oxygen dilution and inspiratory nasopharyngeal resistance, a moderate positive airway pressure effect that may generate alveolar recruitment and an overall greater tolerance and comfort with the interface and the heated and humidified inspired gases.

Conventional oxygen therapy limits the flow of administered oxygen to 15 L/min and is normally administered under non-ideal conditions of temperature and humidity. This limitation of the administered flow means that there is a dilution of the administered oxygen with the ambient air, conditioned by the patient's inspiratory flow peak. Therefore, the higher the inspiratory flow peak, the greater the dilution, which decreases the real FiO_2 supplied to the patient [2,4]. This situation, with little clinical translation in patients with mild hypoxemia, implies that, in patients with severe AKI who present significant hypoxemia and who have inspiratory flow peaks greater than 30L/min, the correction of AKI may not be sufficient by means of oxygen therapy. conventional. An alternative that would solve these limitations of conventional oxygen therapy is the use of non-invasive mechanical ventilation (NIV) devices, although the main limitation of these devices is discomfort and poor patient tolerance [6].

A recent alternative is high-flow oxygen therapy (HFO) [6], which allows a gas flow of up to 60L/min to be supplied through silicone nasal cannulas, with the supplied gas conditioned at the ideal temperature and humidity level (37°C and 100% relative humidity). In addition, the use of HFO allows better management of respiratory secretions, a fact that could be of special importance in patients with ARF of infectious etiology.

In summary, in patients with severe ARF, the use of HFO could allow a rapid improvement in dyspnea, an improvement in hypoxemia, better management of respiratory secretions, and a decreased need for mechanical ventilation.

Oxygen Therapy during Invasive Procedures

During invasive procedures, such as fiberoptic bronchoscopy, it is common for hypoxemia to worsen in relation to the hypoventilation that occurs and the use of sedatives. This worsening of hypoxemia may be even greater if bronchoalveolar lavage is performed and may persist for several hours after the examination. The use of HFO has shown beneficial effects in terms of less worsening of hypoxemia and comfort when compared to conventional oxygen therapy. Recently, a lower degree of hypoxemia has been shown during fiberoptic bronchoscopy in favor of NIV in patients with severe hypoxemia; however, the tolerance and well-being of these patients continued to be much better with the use of HFO [7]. Similarly, the use of HFO should also be considered when performing other invasive procedures, such as transesophageal echocardiography or digestive endoscopy.

Palliative Care

In a randomized feasibility trial, Nava and colleagues recruited 200 patients with solid tumors and acute respiratory failure and limited life expectancy. The study showed a clear decrease in Borg dyspnea score in the NIV group, along with lower requirement of total dose of morphine in the first 48 hrs. Adverse events leading to NIV discontinuation were mainly related to mask intolerance and anxiety [8].

In patients in whom IMV is not indicated, the use of HFO could be beneficial since this device allows a decrease in dyspneic sensation and an improvement in hypoxemia and cough with good tolerance by patients. and that allows them to communicate and even feed themselves.

Chest Trauma

Patients with severe chest trauma often require mechanical ventilation. Only two randomized studies have been conducted [9, 10] comparing NIV with epidural analgesia and conventional mechanical ventilation, and they show that the use of NIV in this subgroup of patients reduces hospital stay and mortality. There are some methodological deficiencies in these studies, since the cases with greater pulmonary involvement were excluded and there is no control group that receives treatment with conventional oxygen therapy. The benefits of NIV in this group have also been demonstrated in several case series.

Based on the existing data, the routine use of NIV cannot be recommended in patients with severe chest trauma in general, although in patients with a stable respiratory situation it can avoid the need for mechanical ventilation.

Keys to Success

The success of NIV in acute respiratory failure depends on numerous factors. The selection of the appropriate patients is crucial. Most of the contraindications for NIV, listed in Table 1, reflect the exclusion criteria in randomized controlled trials, which implies that rather than contraindications they are situations for which NIV has not been proven. Although clinical judgment is important in decision making, the use of predictive factors can also be helpful. Improvement in arterial blood gases and sensorium status, or the response of a set of clinical and physiological parameters within the first and second hours of NIV are used as predictors of success or failure in COPD patients [11].

Table 1. Contraindications of NIV

1. Cardio-respiratory arrest severe encephalopathy
2. Severe gastrointestinal bleeding
3. Severe hemodynamic instability with or without unstable angina
4. surgery or facial trauma
5. upper airway obstruction
6. inability to protect the airway with risk of aspiration or not
7. inability to control secretions

The lack of improvement in these predictive factors, as well as the presence of contraindications (Table 1), can also be considered as criteria for the interruption of NIV and intubation or reintubation. Another issue in evaluating the probable outcome of NIV is colonization of the airway with non-fermenting gram-negative bacilli, the presence of which is notably associated with failure [11]. However, even with a good initial response, patients with COPD with severe AKI treated with NIV may deteriorate later (after more than 48 hours) and frequently require STI.

Weaning

NIV reduces respiratory muscle fatigue and improves ventilation. Its usage has increased during acute settings. Sometimes, patients having COPD, OSA, various neuromuscular disorders including critical illness myoneuropathy require NIV for prolong period. Weaning from NIV in these patients is a difficult and tedious job. Weaning needs to be started only when primary condition is better, and patient meets the clinical criteria shown in Table 2.

Table 2. Clinical criteria to be met by patients before weaning is attempted

	Measure	Character
1.	Arterial pH	≥ 7.35
2.	SpO_2	$> 90\%$
3.	Respiratory rate	≤ 25 / min
4.	Heart rate	≤ 120 / min
5.	Systolic blood pressure	≥ 90 mmHg
6.	Signs of respiratory distress	No agitation, diaphoresis, anxiety

Weaning Strategies

Varied strategies for weaning from NIV has been described:

1. Stepwise reduction in NIV duration.
2. Stepwise reduction in NIV pressure support.
3. Immediate withdrawal of NIV after stabilization.

Regarding HFO therapy, it is difficult to establish guidelines for the fate of HFO and its replacement by a conventional oxygen therapy system. However, it would seem reasonable to decrease FiO_2 first and then flow [6]. A recommendation could be acceptable to maintain the administered flow until correct oxygenation is achieved with FiO_2 less than 0.5. The reduction in flow should be slow (5L/min every 6-8h). Finally, when we obtain correct oxygenation with 20L/min or less and with FiO_2 less than 0.5, we consider replacing the HFO with a conventional oxygen therapy system [5,6]. However, in some patients it is necessary to use HFO intermittently during the weaning phase.

Conclusion

The success of NIV in AKI depends on numerous factors. The selection of the appropriate patients is crucial. Most of the contraindications for NIV, reflect the exclusion criteria in randomized controlled trials, implying that rather than contraindications they are situations for which NIV has not been proven [11]. Although the criteria are important in decision making, the use of predictive factors can also be useful.

Improvement in arterial blood gases and sensorium status, or the response of a set of clinical and physiological parameters within the first and second hours of NIV are used as predictors of success or failure in COPD patients. The lack of improvement in these predictive factors, as well as the presence of contraindications, can also be considered as criteria for discontinuation of NIV and intubation or reintubation. Another issue in evaluating the likely outcome of NIV is colonization of the airway with nonfermenting gram-negative bacilli, the presence of which is strongly associated with failure [4, 5]. However, even with a good initial response, COPD patients with AKI treated with NIV may deteriorate later (after more than 48 hours) and frequently require STI.

The clinical management of acute respiratory failure in adult and pediatric-neonatal patients must take into account the heterogeneity of the clinical scenarios with respect to the indications, stratification, and follow-up for the use of non-invasive ventilation and high-flow therapy with nasal cannula.

Non-invasive ventilation plays a significant role in the management of respiratory failure in acute care hospitals. Its use to treat acute respiratory failure related to COPD exacerbations, cardiogenic pulmonary edema, and patients in immunocompromised states has gained wide acceptance. Many other potential applications are being investigated further. Also, because intensive care units are often full, the use of this technique in other settings is becoming common in many hospitals, but patients must be carefully selected to ensure safety. We expect increased use of non-invasive ventilation as new applications are explored and caregivers develop skills in the technique, but caution should be exercised to restrict use to appropriate applications (i.e., avoid patients with contraindications or excessive delays in invasive ventilation and endotracheal intubation). There is a lot of variability between institutions in how often, how and in what setting this technique is applied and efforts should be made to ensure that skill acquisition helps reduce these differences.

The HFO is a new oxygen therapy option that, through heating and humidification, allows the administration of fully conditioned gas at very high flows, improving oxygenation and patient well-being, and minimizing adverse effects on structures. Nasopharyngeal. Based on current evidence, HFO is an attractive and useful therapeutic option in patients with AKI, as it improves oxygenation, decreases work of breathing, and improves patient well-being. However, more studies are needed to determine its possible impact in terms of morbidity and mortality and cost-effectiveness.

References

[1] Kallstrom T J. American Asociation for Respiratory Care [AARC]. Clinical Practice Guideline: Oxygen therapy for adults in the acute care facitity-2002 revision & update. *Respir. Care* 2002,47; 717-20.

[2] Ferreyro B L, Angriman F, Munshi L, Ferguson N D, Ryus M J, Del Sorbo L, Rochwerg Bram, Saskin R, Wunsch Hannah, Da Costa B R, Scales D C. Association of noninvasive oxygenation strategies with all-cause mortality in adults with acute hypoxemic. Respiratory failure. *JAMA* 2020, 324:57.

[3] Luya C-E, Bouadma L, Morris A C, Dhanani JA, Kollef M, Lipman J, Martin-Loeches I, Nseir S, Ranzani OT, Roquilly A, Schmidt M, Torres A, Timsit JF. Pulmonary infections complicating ARDS. *Intensive Care. Med* 2020;46:2168-2183.

[4] Slutsky A S, Ranieri V M. Ventilator-induced lung injury. *N. Engl. J. Med.* 2013; 369:2126-2136.

[5] Barbe F, Togores B, Rubi M. Noninvasive ventilatory support does not facilitate recovery from acute respiratory failure in chronic obstructive pulmonary disease. *Eur. Respir. J.* 1996;9:1240-1245.

[6] Roca O, Riera F, Torres J, Masclans R. High-Flow oxygen therapy in acute respiratory failure. *Respir. Care.* 53 (2020), pp 408-413.

[7] Simon M, Braurre S, Frings D, Wiontzek A, Klose H, Kluge S. High-Flow nasal cannula oxygen versus Non-invasive ventilation in patients with acute hypoxaemic respiratory failure undergoing flexible bronchoscopy. *A Prospective Randomized Trial.* 18 [2014], pp. 712.

[8] Nava S, Ferrer M, Esquinas A, Sala R, Groff P, Cosentini R, Davide G, Ching-Hsiung L, Cuomo AM, Grassi M. Palliative use of Non-invasive ventilation in end-of-life patients with solid tumors: a randomized feasibility trial. *Lancet Oncol.* 2013; 14[3]: 219-227.

[9] Bolliger C. T, Van Eeden S. F. Treatment of multiple rib fractures. Randomized controlled trial comparing ventilatory with non ventilatory management. *Chest,* 97 [1990],

[10] Gundez M, Unlugerg H, Oralevil M, Iraduoglu K, Akman H. A comparative study of continuous positive airway pressure [CPAP] and intermittent positive pressure ventilation in patients with flail chest. *Emerg. Med. J.* 22 [2005], pp.325-329.

[11] Gaudry S, Messika J, Ricard J-D, Guillo S, Pasquet B, Dubief E, Boukertouta T, Dreyfuss D, Tubach F . Patient-important outcomes in randomized controlled trials in critically ill patients: a systematic review. *Ann. Intensive Care.* 2017;7:28 10.1186/s13613-017-0243-z .

Index

A

B

N

O

P

Q

R

S

T

U

V

W

Editors' Contact Information

Antonio M. Esquinas, M.D, Ph.D, FCCP, FNIV, International Fellow AARC

Intensive Care Unit,
Hospital Morales Meseguer,
Murcia, Spain
antmesquinas@gmail.com

Dimitrios A. Lagonidis MD, PHD, FCCP

Plmonologist-Intensivist
Director of ICU
Critical Care, Pulmonary and Sleep Medicine Services,
Giannitsa General Hospital,
Giannitsa, Greece
lagonidis@gmail.com

Pedro Silva Santos, MD

Pulmonology Unit
Coimbra Hospital and University Center,
Coimbra University Hospitals,
Coimbra, Portugal
pedrorssantos@gmail.com

Bushra Mina, MD, FCCP, FCCM, FACP, FNIV

Pulmonary Critical Care Medicine,
Northwell/Lenox Hill Hospital,
New York, New York, USA
bmina@mindspring.com